healthy
pregnancy

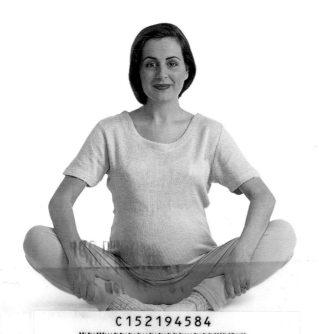

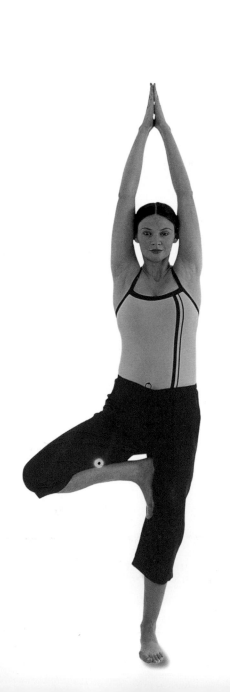

healthy
pregnancy

a practical guide to diet, exercise and relaxation

Gill Thorn

hamlyn

contents

First published in Great Britain
in 2003 by Hamlyn, a division
of Octopus Publishing Group Ltd
2–4 Heron Quays, London E14 4JP

Copyright © Octopus Publishing
Group Ltd 2003

ISBN 0 600 60666 X

A CIP catalogue record for this book is
available from the British Library

Printed and bound in China

10 9 8 7 6 5 4 3 2 1

Safety Note: All reasonable care has
been taken in the preparation of this
book but it is always advisable to
check with your doctor before
embarking on any exercise or diet
programme. This book should not be
considered a replacement for
professional medical treatment; a
physician should be consulted in all
matters relating to health, particularly in
respect of pregnancy and any
symptoms which may require diagnosis
or medical attention. While the advice
and information in this book is
believed to be accurate and the step-by-
step instructions have been devised to
avoid strain, neither the author nor
publisher can accept any legal
responsibility for any injury or illness
sustained while following the exercises,
treatments and diet plan.

Introduction

Adjusting emotionally and physically to having a baby does not happen overnight. The changes that pregnancy brings are exciting, daunting and often a mixture of both, so even if you are thrilled to be pregnant it can take a few weeks to get used to your new situation.

Everyone feels better when their general health is good and they are moderately fit, and pregnant mums are no exception. You do not need to be super-fit when you have a baby, but your body undergoes considerable changes throughout this time and if you are reasonably fit you will cope more easily with the experience.

There are many ways to get fit for birth. Exercise forms part of any regime, but the 9 months you spend in waiting is also an ideal time to give your whole lifestyle some attention, so that you can enjoy your pregnancy to the full.

Checking your diet, reducing your intake of coffee and alcohol, and cutting down on late nights and exposure to smoke-filled rooms will all help to give your baby the best start in life. Balancing the demands of work, family and other commitments may mean you enjoy life more when you are pregnant; learning to relax or use complementary therapies can help you wind down.

In the first 3 months of pregnancy, when your baby's organs are forming, a lot happens but very little shows, so make allowances for the hidden hormone activity if you feel emotional or under the weather. Months 4 to 6 are usually calmer – most women feel well.

Somewhere between 16 and 22 weeks into pregnancy you will feel your baby move – an exciting milestone. Your relationship with your partner and your sex life (possibly on hold, if you

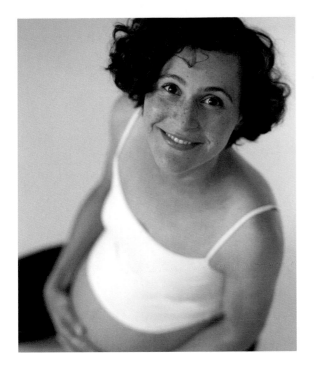

Left *If you are reasonably fit and healthy, you are more likely to enjoy pregnancy and cope more easily with your changing body.*

felt ill earlier in your pregnancy) may improve, and if the idea of a baby was unsettling you may feel more confident. These middle months are a good time to finish projects, plan a holiday or make a real effort to get more exercise.

In the last 3 months of pregnancy you will be larger and heavier. If this is your first baby, you may have some mixed feelings about giving up work; but with the excitement of knowing that your baby will soon be here, this phase of final preparations can be enjoyable.

First baby or not, most women worry about how they will cope with the changes ahead, but if you are fit for birth, in the widest sense, you will feel good, carry your baby more comfortably and give birth more easily. I hope this book will help.

Enjoy your pregnancy!

fitness

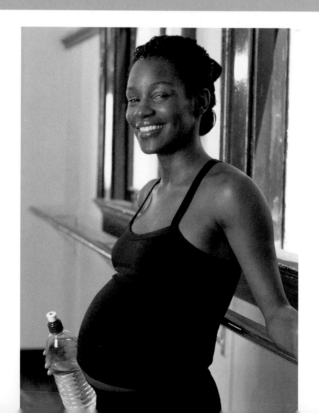

1

- The body miracle

- Feeling good

- Fitness benefits

- Working pregnancy

The body miracle

During pregnancy, your body has the extra task of growing your baby. Enormous changes take place over the 9 months that it takes for a single cell – smaller and lighter than a grain of sand – to grow into a fully functioning baby weighing around 3–3.5kg (7–8lb).

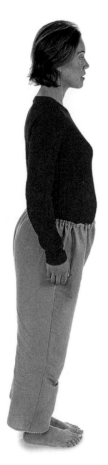

Above At 4 months pregnant.

Hormones

Hormones act on your whole body, and the discomforts they cause are linked to their benefits. They:
- Soften your ligaments, so that your skeleton and your organs adjust their positions to make room for your baby.
- Modify your digestion, so that you absorb nutrients more effectively.
- Lower your metabolic rate, to make your body more energy efficient.

In addition to these changes, your blood volume increases, and to cope with this hormones relax your artery and vein walls and your blood pressure drops a little.

Other changes

The changes in your metabolic rate and the extra blood circulating around your body may make you feel as if you have built-in central heating, especially in your hands and feet. However, your thyroid gland becomes more active and you perspire more freely to regulate your temperature and protect your baby from overheating.

Your heart, lungs and kidneys process waste products and your bladder eliminates water more actively. Your lungs provide oxygen for all the extra blood that is circulating, so your chest cavity enlarges, but you breathe more deeply, rather than faster, so you may find that you are still short of breath when exercising.

At the end of pregnancy your uterus is about a thousand times bigger and weighs 20 times as much as it did at conception. Although you may feel that you are huge, only about half of the expansion is visible from outside your body: the rest takes up space that would otherwise be available for your internal organs.

All these changes put extra stress on your system. You need more rest in the early weeks, when your hormones are fluctuating, and again towards the end, to make up for carrying the extra weight and for lack of sleep.

If you are in good shape, however, you are likely to take it all in your stride, and you will find that your life will go on much as usual unchanged. Relatively small adjustments to your lifestyle, diet or exercise habits can make a big difference to how you feel.

To help to pace a busy lifestyle, for example, you could take a rest for half an hour in your lunch break, or sit with your feet up at regular intervals during the day to read a story, perhaps to one of your other children. If your job is sedentary, you could go for a walk in your lunch break, or make a point of climbing the stairs instead of taking the lift every day.

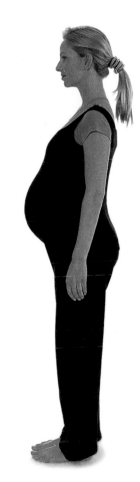

Above At 8 months pregnant.

Feeling good

At the upper end of the fitness scale is the highly trained athlete; at the lower end of the scale is the couch potato who cannot run for a bus or climb a flight of stairs without becoming puffed out. Most women are somewhere in between: fit enough to cope with their normal work, carry out their daily chores and deal with an emergency, but with room for improvement!

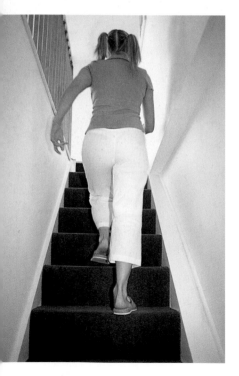

Above Strengthen your buttock muscles, even before pregnancy, by climbing the stairs regularly.

The physical changes of pregnancy and the act of giving birth test your body. When you are fit, you have a feeling of wellbeing and energy. You move flexibly, your body functions effectively and it throws off minor infections easily.

You can judge your own fitness level by your zest for life, your ability to carry out a physical task with the minimum of effort, and your normal energy levels – regardless of your month of pregnancy. The better you feel, the greater the likelihood of your pregnancy and birth being straightforward.

You may also avoid some of the discomforts that are often thought to be simply part of being pregnant, but that are actually affected by your general fitness and the way you use your body. For example:

- Weak buttock and abdominal muscles contribute to backache.
- Slouching instead of standing up straight puts extra pressure on your stomach valve and increases heartburn.
- Poor circulation increases the likelihood of you suffering from cramp and varicose veins.

It may not be possible to avoid all of these discomforts, but women who are generally fit suffer from fewer of them.

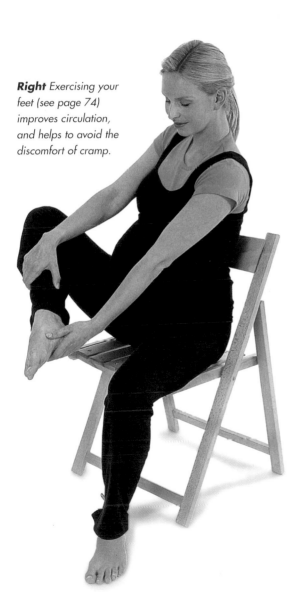

Right Exercising your feet (see page 74) improves circulation, and helps to avoid the discomfort of cramp.

'As soon as I knew I was pregnant I took myself in hand, because I wanted to get the most out of the experience. I looked at my diet and the amount of exercise that I took – very little, as it happens! My partner and I discussed our lifestyle and we decided to make a conscious effort to relax more. Pregnancy provided the incentive to take stock of the balance in our life, and the benefits were immediate and obvious.

'If you feel good you get a new spring in your step and the special months are more enjoyable. Pregnancy has been a beautiful experience. We have kept a journal, taking photos every month and writing something to remind us what it was like. I've kept scan pictures and everything, as a record for the future.'

Anna (42), 8 months pregnant

Fitness benefits

The main elements of fitness are strength, stamina and suppleness, together with a degree of speed and skill. When all these elements are combined you feel good, have plenty of energy and are able to carry out daily tasks efficiently.

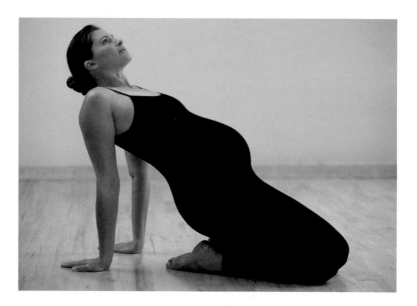

Above *When all the elements of fitness are combined, you are likely to feel good while pregnant.*

Opposite *Having a strong and supple body means everyday tasks are easier to carry out during pregnancy.*

Elements of fitness

Strength. Strong muscles enable you to carry out daily activities such as lifting a toddler or a shopping bag or pushing a supermarket trolley. Strength makes getting up from a low seat easier, protects you from injury, and enables you to respond to sudden emergencies, such as jumping out of the way of a car.

Stamina. Any task that involves repetitive movements or sustained effort requires stamina, which in turn depends on efficient lungs, heart, blood circulation and muscles. Stamina makes it easier to redecorate an entire room, walk briskly when you are late for an appointment or handle a slow labour without getting tired.

Suppleness. If your range of movement is restricted, simple tasks that involve reaching or twisting – such as getting in and out of a car or putting a toddler in a highchair – are more difficult. Suppleness helps to protect you from injury when you carry out awkward jobs around the house or turn suddenly, and it enables you to be comfortable in positions that make giving birth easier.

Skill and speed. The more you do something, the easier it becomes. Skill is needed to carry out basic everyday tasks; speed enables you to run up and down stairs, grab a child who runs out into the road or catch a plate before it smashes on the floor. Although they are not major elements of fitness, these factors contribute to your body's overall efficiency when performing a task.

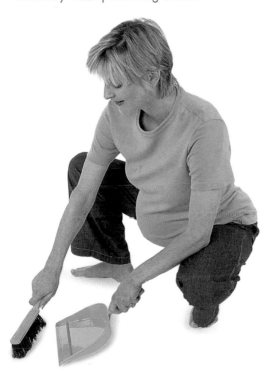

How fit are you?

If you answer 'yes' to any of the following questions, you may want to concentrate on improving the suggested elements of your fitness.

- Do you find it difficult to get out of an armchair or the bath?
  - *leg/arm strength*
  - *suppleness*

- Do you feel breathless if you walk briskly?
  - *stamina*

- Do your legs ache when you climb stairs?
  - *leg strength*
  - *stamina*

- Do you find it difficult to bend down to pick up something?
  - *suppleness*

- Are you exhausted at the end of the day?
  - *strength*
  - *stamina*
  - *suppleness*

Working pregnancy

Working during pregnancy is easier if you get to know what your body needs and you are able to pace yourself. Most women work throughout pregnancy, unless they are ill or their job is dangerous (for example, it involves potentially hazardous chemicals), but they vary in what they can tolerate at different stages. If your job is demanding, it may be difficult to carry on as usual.

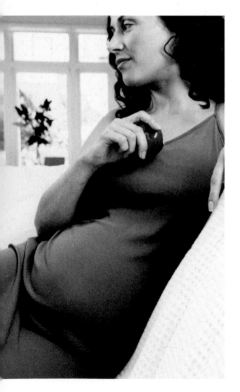

Above Take time to rest when you come home from work.

Having a baby does make a difference. There is no need to feel that it is a personal indulgence and you have to act as though you were not pregnant. Your child will become one of the workers who helps to support your colleagues when they retire, so ask for help when you need it without feeling embarrassed. Ask for a chair or a drink of water. Ask to have a window opened. Ask your employer to move you to a job that is less strenuous, or one in which you can sit down if necessary, or one that involves less travelling.

Know your body

Many women feel tired, sick or emotional during the first 3 months of pregnancy when most of the physical changes are hidden, but you can often reduce stress and carry on working more easily simply by adjusting your lifestyle.

- Eat regularly to keep up your blood sugar level. Choose plenty of carbohydrate foods (see pages 32–33), eating little and often.
- Rest after lunch – at your desk, in the restroom, in your car, in bed.
- Delegate diligently! Other people are often willing to do things if you ask.
- Refuse social invitations temporarily.

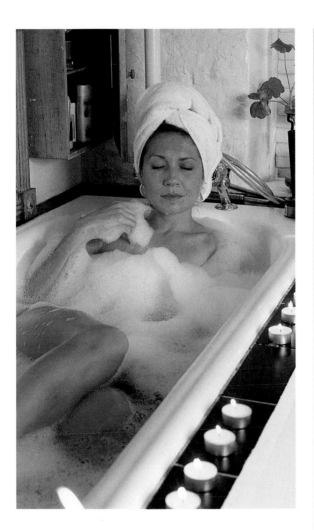

'When I was working I kept going through most of my lunch hour, because I knew if I sat down I wouldn't want to get up again! I hated asking for help, as I felt it made extra work for other people.

'It took me a long time to realize there was really no need to carry on as though I wasn't pregnant. Most people understood and were sympathetic when I tried to leave on time after work as I was absolutely shattered, especially when someone they knew had recently had a baby.

'As soon as I got home I had something to eat, then slept for an hour. Now I'm on maternity leave I plan my day around activity and rest. I have more energy in the morning and the evening, so I make the most of those times and put my feet up in the afternoon.'

Abi (29), 8 months pregnant

- Buy easily prepared convenience foods.
- I luve two or three early nights every week.
- Relax for at least half an hour in the bath, adding lavender aromatherapy oil to the water.
- Have your main meal at lunchtime, so that you only have to prepare a snack in the evening; or ask your partner to prepare the meal.
- Schedule your evening meal so that you can get to bed earlier.

Above left *Relaxing in a bath at the end of the day helps to reduce stress.*

lifestyle

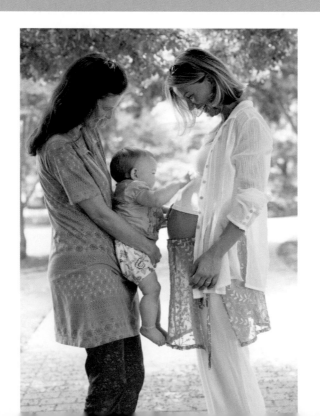

2

- Alcohol

- Medication

- Smoking

- Other hazards

Alcohol

The risks to your baby during pregnancy are tiny compared to those women faced a hundred years ago, when they were poorly nourished and overworked, and medical care was primitive. These days more is known about what causes problems for babies during pregnancy, so it is sensible to reduce or avoid risks wherever possible.

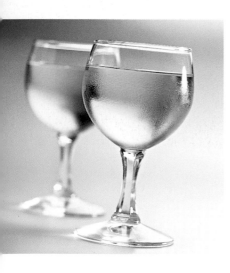

Above Limiting your alcohol intake during pregnancy will reduce the risk to your baby.

It may seem that pregnancy is one long list of things you must not do for the sake of your unborn baby, but if your lifestyle is generally healthy and you take a sensible approach to risk without becoming obsessive, you will know you have done your best. Taking a look at your overall lifestyle is part of getting fit for birth.

Limiting intake

If you drink heavily during pregnancy, you double your risk of miscarriage and increase the chances of having a baby with a major abnormality. The risks start to rise at the equivalent of four measures of spirits or glasses of wine, or two pints of beer or cider per day, increasing steeply at about three times these amounts.

For reasons that are unknown, babies of women over the age of 35 fare worse than those of younger women, and black babies are seven times more vulnerable than white ones, possibly for genetic reasons.

Statistically, you are no more likely to have a baby suffering from foetal alcohol syndrome if you have a glass or two of wine each week, or even one each day, than if you abstain entirely; but alcohol-related risks are greater if you drink heavily

5 ways to reduce alcohol consumption

1 Drink alcohol only on certain days and choose fruit juices on the other days.

2 Adopt the French habit of diluting your wine with mineral water.

3 On social occasions, stick to one glass of wine and drink it slowly.

4 Choose low-alcohol drinks for preference, but check the bottle – some lemonade- or fruit-based drinks contain more alcohol than you might think.

5 Ask for long drinks rather than shorts and make them last.

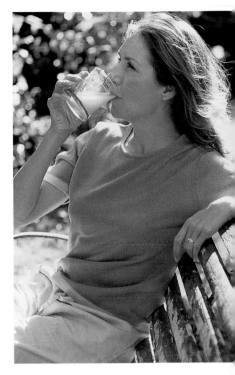

Above *Choosing to drink fruit juice instead of alcohol on certain days will reduce your overall consumption.*

on most days, or your diet is poor, or if you smoke. Consuming enough alcohol to feel drunk in a short time also increases the risk.

However, individuals respond differently to alcohol, so it is impossible to state that a particular limit is safe or otherwise: what is fine for one person may be damaging for another. If you think you may have a drink problem, tackle it as soon as possible, and preferably before you become pregnant.

Many women prefer to cut out alcohol completely during pregnancy, instead of reducing the amount they drink. This is easy once people know that you are pregnant (indeed, the alcohol police may reaise eyebrows as soon as you have a noticeable bump). During the first three months you could dream up a plausible excuse, or enlist your partner's help if you want to keep your pregnancy a secret.

Medication

All drugs alter your body chemistry, so treat them with great caution around the time of conception and during pregnancy. Check with your doctor, pharmacist or a qualified alternative practitioner before taking any medication that is not essential to your health.

'I take steroid tablets for asthma and my doctor has advised me to continue, because poorly controlled asthma is linked with problems like slow foetal growth. My pattern of attacks hasn't changed, but I treat every attack promptly to make sure that the baby gets plenty of oxygen.

'When I was expecting Finlay I improved my stamina by walking, and I didn't have any problem with asthma during labour because the body produces extra cortisone and adrenalin which give natural protection. In this pregnancy I feel generally fitter because I'm running around after a toddler all day.'

Marie (24), mother of Finlay (2) and 20 weeks pregnant

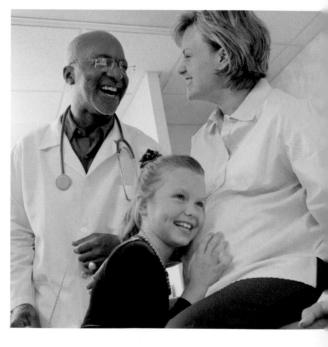

This warning includes over-the-counter remedies for minor ailments such as colds and 'flu; aromatherapy oils, which are absorbed through the skin and can have powerful effects; herbal or homeopathic remedies (see pages 90–91); and vitamin or slimming pills (see pages 36–37).

Over-the-counter remedies for self-limiting conditions often contain a mix of ingredients, some of which may not be suitable for use during pregnancy. Certain herbs and aromatherapy oils can be beneficial during pregnancy or labour, but others are contra-indicated. To be on the safe side, make no assumptions – check with an expert.

If you have a condition that needs regular medication (including asthma if you use an inhaler), tell your doctor that you plan to become pregnant, or discuss it as soon as possible during pregnancy.

Your medication may have no known problems, or there may be an alternative treatment approach that can be tried. If your condition requires treatment with drugs that could pose hazards, talking it through with an expert will help you to decide what to do.

Recreational drugs

Street drugs are known to increase the risks of abnormality, miscarriage and poor foetal growth.
Ecstasy is an amphetamine derivative that has been linked with cleft palate and heart problems.
Marijuana and cannabis have been linked with premature birth.
Cocaine increases the likelihood of abnormality, bleeding and premature birth; it constricts blood vessels and reduces the baby's oxygen supply.
Heroin increases the risk of premature labour and low birth weight, and trebles the risk of miscarriage or stillbirth. Sudden withdrawal during pregnancy can cause miscarriage or premature labour.

If you are addicted to any street drug, it is important to seek help before conceiving or as soon as possible during pregnancy. People offering rehabilitation do not judge their clients and the programmes tend to be especially effective when you are well motivated. Thinking about your baby's future may give you this incentive.

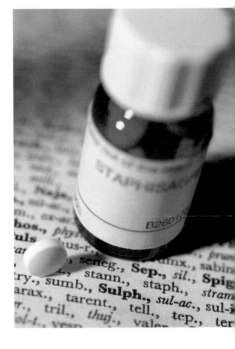

Above If you are taking any medication, homeopathic or otherwise, check with a qualified practitioner that it is safe to take during pregnancy.

Opposite Talk to a doctor if you need to take regular medication.

Smoking

Women who find it hard to give up smoking often feel both guilty and lacking in willpower – but do keep trying. For every cigarette that remains unsmoked, your baby escapes a dose of nicotine and carbon monoxide.

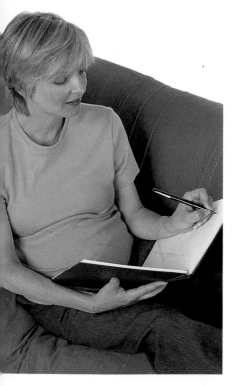

Above Keep a diary of your smoking habits if you want to give up gradually.

Smoking during pregnancy is associated with more miscarriages, vaginal bleeding, premature births and low birth-weight babies. If you are over 35, there is also a significant increase in the risk of your baby having a minor malformation and five times the risk of low birth weight (a major cause of infant illness) compared to a younger smoker.

Even if you have smoked for many years, if you stop before you conceive your baby has the same chance of good health as a non-smoker's baby. In early pregnancy nausea often makes giving up easier, and if you quit before month 4 of pregnancy you protect your baby from the worst effects of smoking, which occur between months 4 and 9. Even quitting in month 9 may make your uterus work more effectively and help to preserve your baby's oxygen flow during labour.

Giving up

If you want to give up slowly, keep a diary of the times at which you smoke each day. When a pattern emerges, distract yourself from the cigarettes that are least important to your routine. Have some early nights so that you are not overtired. Use the money you save for some treats as a reward.

However, more people succeed by stopping completely than by cutting down. Heavy smokers say that the worst craving lasts for a couple of weeks and some women find the following distractions helpful when they crave a cigarette:

- Relax your shoulders and take a few deep breaths, pausing between each one. Turn your attention to visualizing a pleasant scene.
- Eat a spoonful of yoghurt, an apple, a stick of celery or a raw carrot – healthier than chocolate or fattening snacks – or chew gum.
- If smoking helped you to concentrate, fiddle with a paper clip, a rubber band, worry beads or a piece of modelling clay.
- Change your routine. Go for a short walk, make a coffee, count to 100.

What else helps?

If you find it hard to give up on your own, there is plenty of help available:

- Books or voluntary groups can offer support, or your doctor may refer you to a local quit group.
- Simply talking to a health professional helps one person in 20 to give up, while the incentive of being pregnant trebles this success rate.
- Chewing gum, inhalers and nasal sprays increase success rates by about 12 per cent, but consult your doctor before trying them.
- Hypnosis or acupuncture, alone or with group therapy, helps some people to quit, although there is no evidence that these treatments work better overall than a placebo.

Pregnancy is a good motivation, however, so even if you have tried before and failed you may find it easier than you expect to give up.

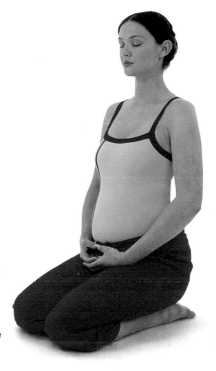

Above To distract yourself from craving a cigarette, try relaxing – see pages 84–87 for further techniques.

Other hazards

You cannot avoid exposure to everything that might possibly prove harmful during pregnancy, but you can use common sense. Most things are probably safe in moderation, so aim to avoid all excess. For example, if you enjoy coffee, have one or two cups of a mild brew every day, not six strong ones.

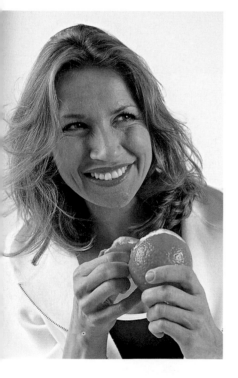

Above Healthy eating can make a big difference to the start you give your baby in life.

The effect of many common products, such as oven cleaners, pest control sprays and hair dyes, are unknown. This does not necessarily mean that they are harmful to an unborn baby, but nor can anyone claim that they are safe. You may want to avoid unnecessary exposure to any chemicals that have toxic warnings on the packaging, or that remind you to keep them off your skin.

Some people may be more susceptible to the effects of chemicals used in crop sprays than others. If you live in a rural area, you may want to ask local farmers to tell you when spraying is due to be carried out so that you can stay indoors.

If a doctor or dentist suggests an X-ray, you could ask whether it is essential. If it is, tell the operator that you are pregnant so that your pelvic area can be shielded to reduce any risks.

Do your best

Great emphasis is placed on avoiding risks during pregnancy, and it can be hard to keep everything in perspective. Life is not perfect; individual genetic factors and advances in modern ways of living will always cause problems for a small number of babies. For many years X-rays were considered safe to an unborn child. We now know they are hazardous; undoubtedly practices considered safe today will be outlawed in fifty years.

Women are often made to feel that it is entirely their responsibility to ensure that their child is healthy, but you cannot control everything, and there is no point in worrying about things you can do nothing about. The best approach is to concentrate on what you can do to give your baby a good start in life: things like avoiding smoking, alcohol and recreational drugs, together with the best possible diet (see Chapter 3), will probably make the biggest difference.

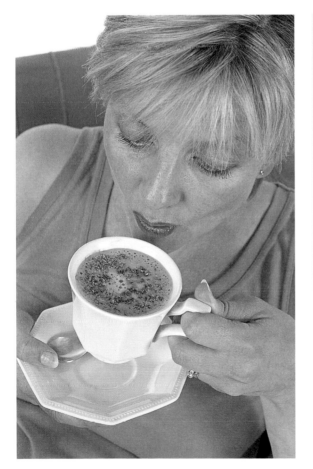

'I worried about everything when I was expecting Jack, but you cannot put things on hold just because you're pregnant so I've decided to avoid what I reasonably can and ignore the rest. I want us all to enjoy ourselves as a family and that means using common sense. Lots of risks are very small and I don't want Jack and Chloe to get the idea that pregnancy stops you doing things that are fun.'

Sue (43), mother of Jack (6) and Chloe (2), and 9 weeks pregnant

Left You can still enjoy coffee, but try drinking only one or two cups of a mild brand each day.

diet and weight

- Healthy eating

- What should you eat?

- Important vitamins and minerals

- Dietary supplements

- Improve your diet

3

- Food precautions

- Body Mass Index

- Average weight gain

- Does your weight matter?

- Weight watching

Healthy eating

A good diet reduces the chances of foetal abnormality and helps to ensure that your baby grows as well as possible. You do not need a super diet, just the normal sort of healthy eating that benefits everybody. This means food rich in vitamins, minerals and fibre, but not too high in sugar or fat.

Fibre is essential for the absorption of nutrients from food and for the process of digestion. It also helps to prevent constipation and haemorrhoids.

Natural sugars such as fructose are present in many wholefoods, but refined sugar adds calories without nutrients.

Ideally, **fat** should provide no more than 30 per cent of your total daily calories, but many products, including some so-called health foods, contain well over this amount. Most of the fat in processed foods, sandwiches and snacks is saturated or hydrogenated. Unsaturated fats, found in things like sunflower or olive oils, fresh nuts and oily fish, are better for you as they contain essential fatty acids. If these are missing from your diet your baby will grow because your body supplies the best substitute available, but development may not be as good as it could be.

How much fat?

The percentage of fat may be openly declared on the packaging of a product if the company is proud of it. If the percentage has not been displayed, you can work it out for yourself: multiply the number of fat grams by 9 (1g fat = 9 calories), then divide by the total number of calories and multiply by 100. If the result is more than 30 per cent, the product is high in fat.

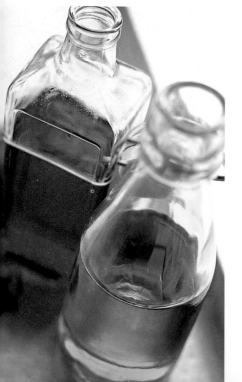

Below Unsaturated fats such as those found in olive oil contain essential fatty acids.

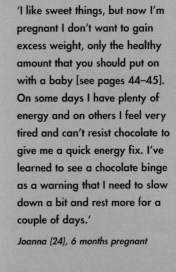

'I like sweet things, but now I'm pregnant I don't want to gain excess weight, only the healthy amount that you should put on with a baby [see pages 44–45]. On some days I have plenty of energy and on others I feel very tired and can't resist chocolate to give me a quick energy fix. I've learned to see a chocolate binge as a warning that I need to slow down a bit and rest more for a couple of days.'

Joanna (24), 6 months pregnant

'Before I was pregnant I ate hardly any fruit and vegetables. It was a real effort at first, but you get used to it. Now I'll choose an apple rather than a packet of crisps – my mum can't believe it, but I do feel better for eating more healthily!'

Lily (21), 37 weeks pregnant

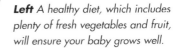

Left *A healthy diet, which includes plenty of fresh vegetables and fruit, will ensure your baby grows well.*

What should you eat?

Everyone has individual nutritional requirements and different diets can be equally healthy, so it is impossible to say exactly what you should eat during pregnancy.

The easiest way to make sure that you eat healthily is to choose a variety of whole, fresh foods, as these contain a range of nutrients that are removed when food is highly processed. Restrict alcohol and fatty or sugary snacks such as crisps, cakes and fizzy drinks to occasional treats – they provide more calories than nutrients. If you need individual advice, ask your doctor to refer you to a nutritionist.

Below You should include a source of protein in your meals to make sure you are eating a balanced diet.

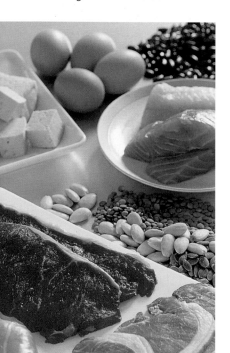

A balanced diet

You should aim to eat a varied diet each day, containing at least:

- 5 portions of fruit and vegetables
- 5 portions of complex carbohydrates
- 5 portions from the protein and fat or dairy produce groups combined

The more variety in the foods you choose, the better.

Q I don't eat much meat or dairy produce and am thinking of cutting them out completely now that I'm pregnant. Is this a good idea?

A A vegetarian or vegan diet can be very healthy, provided you make sure it is balanced. If you cut out meat and dairy produce you need to replace them with other sources of protein such as pulses and nuts. You also need to make sure you get enough vitamin B12 and iron. Ask your doctor to refer you to a nutritionist who will be able to advise you.

Food group pyramid

The pyramid diagram below shows, proportionally, how much of the following food groups you should be eating every day.

❶ Fats
Olive, sunflower, safflower, walnut oils

❷ Dairy produce
Milk, butter, cheese and yoghurt

❸ Proteins
Meat, pulses, nuts, eggs, white and oily fish, seeds, butter and yoghurt

❹ Vegetables
Carrots, broccoli, beans, cabbage, cauliflower, parsnips, mushrooms, spinach, brussels sprouts, onions, leeks, celery and lettuce

❺ Fruit
Tomatoes, apples, pears, citrus fruit and soft fruit

❻ Complex carbohydrates
Wholemeal bread, pasta, rice, potatoes, buckwheat, couscous, pitta bread, noodles and pizza bases

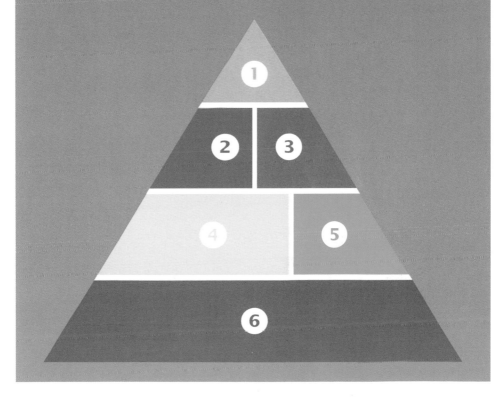

Important vitamins and minerals

Vitamin A
What it does Promotes bone growth and healthy eyes, skin and gums; helps mucous membranes to resist irritation and infections
Found in Carrots, green leafy vegetables, broccoli, milk, cheese, salmon, halibut, apricots, peaches

Vitamin B-complex
What it does Promotes healthy nervous system, tissues and skin; helps to produce red blood cells and metabolize carbohydrates, fats and proteins to release energy
Found in Red meat, yeast extract, dairy produce, eggs, nuts, bananas, pulses, wholemeal bread, fish, rice, bran, potatoes and beans

Vitamin C
What it does Promotes healthy skin, bones and joints; increases the absorption of iron; helps the body to recover from stress; fights infection
Found in Citrus fruits, blackcurrants, green peppers, broccoli, cabbage, potatoes

Vitamin D
What it does Promotes strong bones and teeth; regulates absorption of phosphorus and calcium
Found in Eggs, dairy produce, margarine, oily fish (herrings, kippers, salmon, mackerel, sardines and tuna); exposure to sunlight also increases vitamin D levels

Vitamin E
What it does Promotes healthy circulatory, nervous and reproductive systems; strengthens muscles, aids stamina and helps lower blood pressure; prevents breakdown of saturated fatty acids to form toxic substances in the digestive tract
Found in Almonds, Brazil nuts, olive, sunflower and safflower oils, eggs, dairy produce, wholegrain cereals, broccoli, carrots, celery, apples, avocados

Vitamin K
What it does Produces blood-clotting substance that prevents haemorrhage
Found in Lean meat, broccoli, spinach, tomatoes, nuts, oatmeal, avocados; also manufactured by bacteria in the gut

Calcium
What it does Strengthens bones and teeth; promotes healthy immune system; helps in muscle contraction, blood clotting, energy production and hormone release
Found in Dairy produce, green leafy vegetables, oranges, bread, sardines, soya, wheatgerm, yeast extract, molasses, raisins, prunes, almonds, Brazil nuts

Iron
What it does Combines with protein to form haemoglobin which carries oxygen around the body; helps in muscle contraction and to prevent fatigue and breathlessness
Found in Red meat, molasses, sardines, dried fruit, asparagus, wholegrains, beans, lentils, almonds, wholemeal bread, cocoa, potatoes, broccoli

Zinc
What it does Essential to over 100 enzymes that process nutrients in the body
Found in Cheddar cheese, oysters, chicken, turkey, lamb, pork, tuna, eggs, peas, carrots, wholemeal bread, sweetcorn, oatmeal, seafoods, wholegrains

Magnesium
What it does Promotes healthy tissues, muscles and nerves; helps in absorption of other nutrients; deficiency may contribute to miscarriage and premature birth
Found in Nuts, seafood, meat, eggs, dairy produce, dried apricots, almonds, brazil nuts, green leafy vegetables, wholegrains, hard drinking water

Dietary supplements

As a general rule, vitamins and minerals are better absorbed and used by the body in the natural combinations present in food. A poor diet plus a pill or a vitamin-fortified drink is *not* the same as a good, balanced diet.

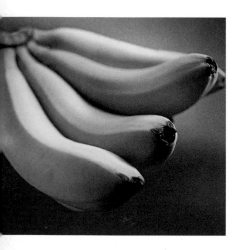

Above *Bananas are a source of folic acid, a B vitamin that is important in the formation of a baby's neural tube.*

However, supplements can be valuable in some circumstances. They may provide a temporary boost if you are unable to eat balanced meals because of your work or travel schedule, if you are recovering from an illness or if you suffer from severe pregnancy sickness.

Check with your doctor or pharmacist before you self-prescribe any vitamin or mineral supplements other than folic acid, as they can interact with other medications. In addition, an excess of some nutrients can be harmful.

Folic acid

This B vitamin is found in dark green leafy vegetables, yeast extract, nuts, eggs, oranges, cheddar cheese, bananas, lettuce, broccoli, brussels sprouts, haddock and salmon. It is important for cell division, reproduction and for the formation of red blood cells. A deficiency prevents the baby's neural tube from forming, which can lead to defects such as spina bifida.

Every woman is advised to take a folic acid supplement (400mcg) for at least 3 months before and after conception, because some women carry a gene that prevents them from using folic acid well even if they eat healthily. There is some evidence that supplements may increase the multiple birth rate slightly; and if you use medication for epilepsy you should consult your doctor before taking them.

Food cravings

If you are poorly nourished your baby will quickly use up your reserves. Cravings for strange things such as chalk may indicate a lack of nutrients, but if you generally eat healthily a passion for chocolate or citrus fruit is more likely to indicate that your body needs energy, or extra vitamin C to counteract symptoms of stress.

Exhaustion makes many women turn to snacks that provide a quick energy boost, but these are often high in sugar and fat and may take away your appetite for healthier food. Getting extra rest is a more effective strategy.

Q I did not realize I was pregnant, so I had no chance to take a folic acid supplement. Could I have harmed my baby?

A Folic acid protects your baby against neural tube defects, so ideally you should take a supplement before and during early pregnancy. However, if you were well nourished before conception your baby will have drawn on your reserves during organ formation and will have an excellent chance of developing normally, especially if you ate plenty of foods like green leafy vegetables that contain folic acid.

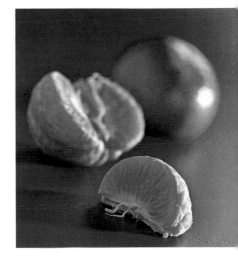

Above If you have a craving for citrus fruit, your body may need an energy boost or extra vitamin C to reduce stress symptoms.

Improve your diet

If you judge your usual diet against the recommendations on pages 30–33, you may be able to see where you could make effective changes. Small adjustments in the foods you choose and the way you serve them can make a big difference.

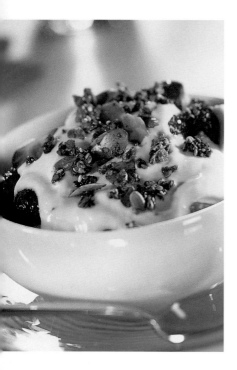

For example, complex carbohydrates give you energy: staples like wholemeal bread, potatoes and brown rice are both filling and full of nutrients, so keep them in stock.

Fresh vegetables tend to lose vitamins and minerals during storage, so either buy them frozen or shop every day or two if you can. Cooking vegetables lightly or, where possible, eating them raw can improve their nutrient value at no extra cost. Whole fish, such as trout or mackerel, are delicious baked in foil, while ready-prepared portions from the freezer can be diced and added to a stir fry instead of meat.

Here are some ways to boost your diet easily:

Breakfast
- Drink some orange juice, or any pure fruit juice.
- Eat half a grapefruit.
- Add a sliced banana to your breakfast cereal.
- Switch from white toast to wholemeal.
- Adopt the French habit of drinking hot chocolate for breakfast instead of coffee or tea.

Lunch
- Eat a salad or some vegetable soup.
- Take sticks of cucumber, celery or carrot in your packed lunch, plus an apple or a banana instead of cake or a chocolate bar.
- Add tomato, lettuce or beansprouts to your sandwiches.

Above *Fresh fruit topped with yoghurt makes a healthy dessert.*

Opposite, above *Remember to drink enough water during the day.*

Opposite, below *At breakfast drink pure fruit juice instead of coffee or tea.*

Top tips

1 Try not to miss a meal, as this can cause your metabolism to fluctuate.

2 Nibbling pieces of raw fruit or vegetables, bite-sized sandwiches or plain dry biscuits can help to reduce nausea in early pregnancy.

3 Instead of having a snack with your toddler or when you get home from work, eat your evening meal earlier.

4 Drink plenty of water to help your system run smoothly.

5 Pasta and potatoes give you more energy and satisfy your hunger for a longer period than sweet things. Chocolate tends to give your blood sugar levels a short-term boost, but when they drop you feel hungry again.

6 If you tend to eat for a quick energy fix, try a few early nights instead, or scale down any extra commitments you have taken on so that you can cope more comfortably.

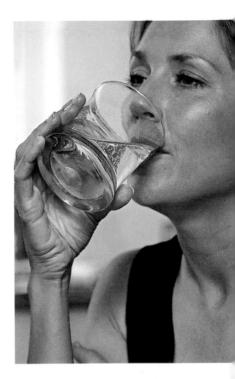

Dinner
- Add a vegetable, such as broccoli or cauliflower, to a casserole or pasta sauce.
- When eating out, order boiled rather than roast potatoes, or extra vegetables instead of chips.
- Eat fresh fruit instead of a pudding.

Snacks
- Eat grapes, cherry tomatoes, celery, carrot sticks or dry-roasted sunflower seeds.
- Dates, raisins or dried apricots make healthy, sweet-tasting snacks.

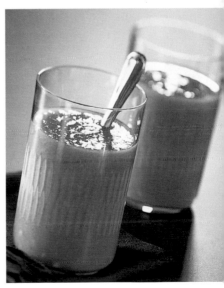

Food precautions

Good kitchen hygiene will help you to avoid potentially damaging infections. Store cooked meat separately from raw meat. Cook food thoroughly, especially if it is being reheated. Wash all fruit and vegetables before eating them and keep the temperature in your refrigerator below 4°C (39°F).

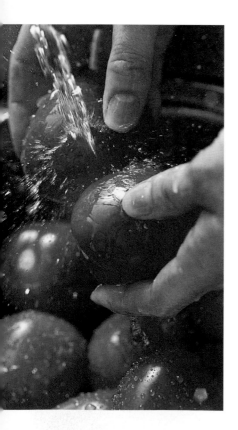

Above It is very important to wash all fruit and vegetables thoroughly before eating them.

Take care

The following foods could potentially cause illnesses, such as listeriosis and toxoplasmosis or other problems, which can be harmful to your baby:

- Cook-chill and ready-prepared foods, such as cooked ham or prepared salads, that could be contaminated before you buy them.
- Soft and blue-veined cheeses.
- Unpasteurized milk or cheese (cow's, sheep's or goat's).
- Soft-boiled and raw eggs (for example, in home-made desserts and mayonnaise).
- Soft-whip ice cream.
- Undercooked meat.
- Liver.
- Pâté (meat, vegetable or fish).
- Shellfish.
- Peanuts.
- Other nuts in large quantities.

'Eating for two'

In early pregnancy your digestion and metabolic rate (the speed at which food is processed and utilized) slow down to increase the absorption of essential nutrients, such as calcium which helps to build strong bones. This ensures that your baby develops well even if you feel sick and cannot eat very much.

After about 16 weeks your metabolism speeds up again, but hormones relax your gut so that the food you eat passes through more slowly and your body continues to absorb nutrients more effectively. This is one of the ways in which your body adapts to the extra demands of pregnancy.

As an example, your body needs more iron to boost the production of red blood cells. Blood plasma, the solution that carries these cells, rises by about 50 per cent during pregnancy; this reduces the proportion of red blood cells available to carry nutrients around your body and provide food and oxygen for your baby. If your diet is healthy, some of the extra iron you need comes from the food you eat (see page 35), but by the end of pregnancy your body is also able to absorb nine times as much iron as usual from your food.

Clever adaptations like this mean that unless you are underweight, expecting twins or have another special reason for eating more than usual, there is no need to 'eat for two' during pregnancy. The quality of the food you eat is more important than the quantity: it should provide nutrients rather than empty calories.

Most women often find that their instinctive appetite is a guide to how much food they need, and they naturally feel hungrier towards the end of their pregnancy.

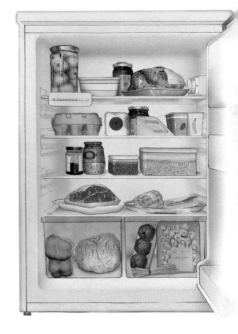

Above *The temperature of your refrigerator should be below 4°C (39°F), and all cooked and raw meat should be covered and kept separately.*

Body Mass Index

The Body Mass Index (BMI) provides a guide to the best weight range for good health when you are not pregnant, regardless of your age or body type. You usually start to gain weight after about 12 weeks of pregnancy, so your midwife will record your BMI at your booking visit, to help her to assess risk.

Slimming diets

Pregnancy is not a good time to go on a diet, as it could make it difficult for your baby to receive enough essential nourishment. Nutrients work together to build a healthy baby: for example, vitamin C helps you to absorb iron and protects your supply of vitamins A and E, but it needs replacing frequently as very little is stored.

Slimming diets put your baby on a diet too, which could lead to poor health or growth. Eating healthily according to your appetite is preferable.

If you are within the normal weight range for your height, you are less likely to suffer problems such as high blood pressure or diabetes during pregnancy. A BMI of 20–25 is ideal for optimum health.

Orange band (BMI under 17) You may have difficulty conceiving. If you are poorly nourished when you become pregnant, your baby may lack nutrients before the placenta is fully developed and able to supply them from your blood.

Yellow band (BMI 17–19) You are a little underweight, but if you gain at a reasonable rate your baby should be fine. If your baby is not growing, you may be weighed over several weeks while you rest more and improve your diet. You may need extra food to make sufficient milk for breastfeeding.

Green band (BMI 20–25) This is the weight range associated with fewest problems.

Blue band (BMI 26–30) You are a little heavy, so are more likely to suffer discomforts such as heartburn, varicose veins, tiredness, breathlessness or skin irritation caused by friction and perspiration.

Purple band (BMI over 30) Women in this band tend to suffer from health problems that can complicate pregnancy, such as high blood pressure and diabetes. Medical procedures such as epidurals and foetal heart monitoring can be more difficult to carry out, and the baby may be slightly heavier than average.

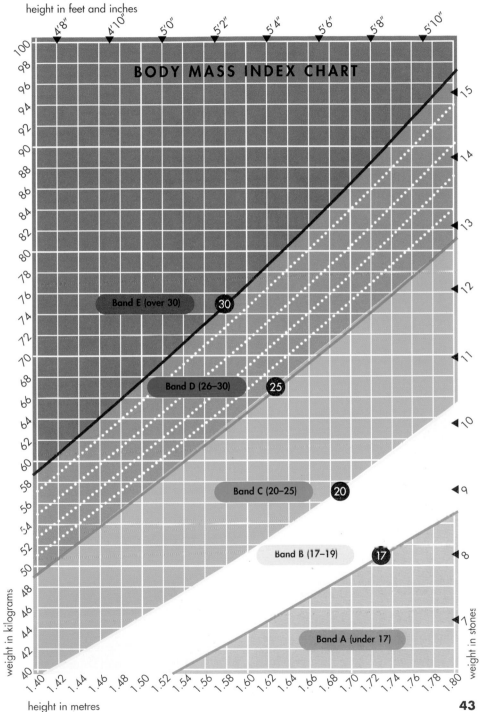

height in feet and inches

BODY MASS INDEX CHART

Band E (over 30)

30

Band D (26–30)

25

Band C (20–25)

20

Band B (17–19)

17

Band A (under 17)

weight in kilograms

weight in stones

height in metres

Average weight gain

Part of the weight you gain during pregnancy is directly associated with the baby, the placenta, extra fluids and so on. The rest consists of the amount of fat you add to your body. Overall weight gain in pregnancy averages 12kg (27lb), but anything between 5 and 15.5kg (11 and 34lb) is considered normal.

'My life used to revolve around diets, so when I was expecting Lucy I felt free to eat what I liked for the first time in years. The more I ate the more I wanted and I put on four or five stones [25–30kg]. My doctor and midwife did not seem concerned, but I felt uncomfortably huge. In this pregnancy I put on no weight for the first 3 months, but now my appetite has returned. I run after Lucy all morning and then eat a healthy salad sandwich, but I avoid cake for lunch because once I start I just can't stop!'

Julie (29), mother of Lucy (2) and 18 weeks pregnant

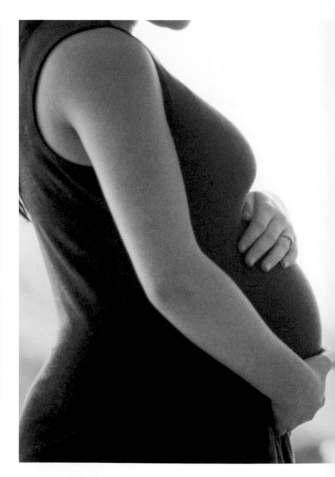

Right *By the end of pregnancy most women have gained about 12kg (27lb) in weight.*

On average, women put on no extra weight in the first 3 months of pregnancy, about 3kg (7lb) in weeks 13–20; another 5.5–6.5kg (12–14lb) in weeks 21–30, and a further 3kg (7lb) in weeks 31–36. In the last month your baby gains weight, but you lose a little because the volume of amniotic and other body fluids fall.

You may put on more weight than average if you are tall and heavily built, if your baby is large or if you are expecting more than one baby. If you have a sedentary job you may not burn off calories as easily as someone who is more active – say, looking after small children.

On average, women expecting their first baby gain an extra 0.9kg (2lb) compared to those on their second or subsequent pregnancies. This may be because they are more likely to have high blood pressure, which tends to be associated with fluid retention, or their metabolism may be less efficient than in later pregnancies.

How total weight gain is made up

Your total weight gain is made up of the baby, the placenta, extra blood and other fluids including amniotic fluid (the water surrounding the baby), the increased weight of your uterus and breasts, plus stores of fat. If you put on no extra fat, you can expect to return to within a kilo (a couple of pounds) of your pre-pregnancy weight 2–3 weeks after giving birth.

Baby	3.3kg	(7½lb)
Placenta	0.7kg	(1½lb)
Amniotic fluid	0.7kg	(1½lb)
Uterus	0.9kg	(2lb)
Breasts	0.5kg	(1lb)
Blood and fluid	2.6kg	(6lb)
Stored fat	3.3kg	(7½lb)
Total	12kg	(27lb)

Does your weight matter?

If you are within the normal weight range when you conceive and you gain steadily as your baby grows, you are likely to be healthier and to suffer fewer problems during pregnancy. It is impossible to say exactly how much weight gain you should aim for: most women put on a kilo or two over and above the gain associated with the pregnancy.

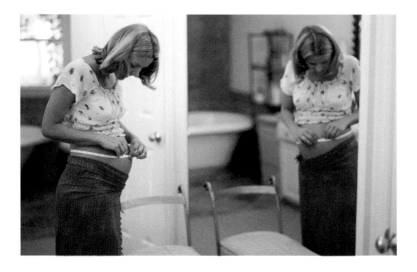

Above If you gain weight steadily as your pregnancy progresses, you will be healthier and find it easier to return to your previous weight several weeks after the birth.

Some women are more energy efficient than others and store large amounts of fat instead of burning it. This was originally a safeguard against food shortages: women who laid down fat were able to survive famine and pass on their genes. Today there is less need for fat stores, although they do provide extra energy for breastfeeding.

In general, doctors cannot tell a normal pregnancy from one that is not just by looking at weight gain or loss, although you may want to

Calorie quiz

1 The average woman needs to consume about 2,000 calories per day when not pregnant. Roughly how many extra calories does she need during pregnancy?

a 200   **b** 450   **c** 550   **d** 950

2 Which of these provide the extra calories she needs?

a Two slices of wholemeal toast with butter or margarine

b A banana and a glass of fruit juice

c A jacket potato with a little cheese

3 Which of these activities burns up the most calories in half an hour?

a Light housework   **b** Swimming lengths

c A brisk walk

Answers

1 a Your body reduces its metabolic rate and becomes more energy efficient during pregnancy, so there are no reasons why you need to eat for two.

2 a, b or c Each provides about 200 calories.

3 b Vigorous, whole-body exercise uses more calories. For example, swimming burns about 230 calories in half an hour, brisk walking about 180 and housework only 60.

discuss a sudden gain with your midwife. Women gain weight at different rates, but you may only be weighed once during pregnancy to establish your Body Mass Index. Excess kilos, however, make pregnancy more uncomfortable.

If you lose weight (or do not gain any after 12 weeks of pregnancy), you may need to eat more or rest more. If the kilos are piling on, fewer calories or more exercise may help. Your gain will be steady if the food you eat balances the energy you use.

Weight watching

Average weight gain in pregnancy is only a guide: the trend is more important than the weekly gain. If you regularly put on more than about 0.5kg (1lb) a week between months 4 and 8, however, you may want to keep an eye on what you eat, or get more exercise.

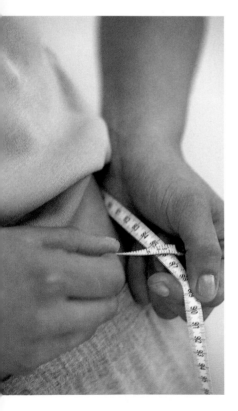

Above Discuss sudden or lack of weight gain with your midwife, who will check all is well.

Your weight tends to regulate naturally if you eat healthily and according to your appetite, provided you do not get so tired that you eat high-calorie snacks for energy.

Guidelines for pregnancy

- If you are in your teens, or you smoke or use street drugs, try to gain towards the upper end of the normal range (say, 13.5–15.5kg/30–34lb). This can boost your baby's birth weight. Low birth-weight babies are more likely to suffer health problems.
- If you cannot keep anything down, or you suffer from anorexia or bulimia, tell your midwife. If you lose weight rapidly you could become under-nourished or dehydrated.
- If you gain nothing for a couple of weeks, or put on 1.5–2kg (3–4lb) and cannot think of a reason (such as a holiday where you ate more than usual), check with your midwife that all is well.
- Tell your midwife if you gain weight rapidly in the last 10 weeks of pregnancy. Fluid retention is often harmless, but could be an early warning sign of pre-eclampsia, a disease of pregnancy.
- Restricting your diet does not help you to have a smaller baby and an easier birth! A poorly nourished baby often suffers retarded growth, which can lead to a more complicated labour.

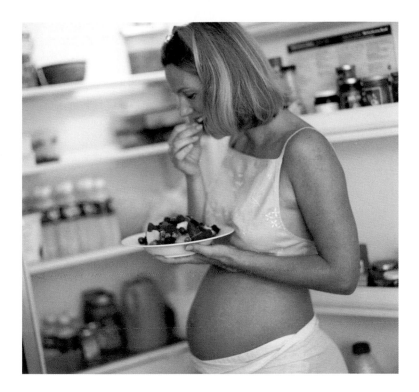

Q I know that I'm overweight and I would like to lose a stone [6.5kg]. How should I set about doing this safely, now that I have the motivation of being pregnant?

A Exercise is a good way to help control your weight. If you want a safe, steady weight loss of 0.5–1kg (1–2lb) per week, increase the amount of exercise you take and cut down slightly on portion sizes. You could walk regularly, gradually increasing the distance and speed (see page 55), or go swimming once or twice a week. Make sure that you get sufficient rest so that you are not tempted to fill up on cake or crisps to give you an energy boost. Make allowances for the pregnancy-related gain; you may want to avoid weighing yourself, as this can be disheartening.

Above Eat plenty of fruit rather than high-calorie snacks, to avoid putting on excess weight during pregnancy.

exercise

- What sort of exercise?

- Where to start

- Exercise safely

- Stretching in pregnancy

- Exercise programme

- Warm up and cool down

4

- Inner thighs and lower back

- Pelvic mobility

- Upper body

- Lower body

- Leg strength

- Circulation and pelvic floor

What sort of exercise?

Most women benefit from gentle, non-competitive exercise while pregnant. It improves fitness, boosts your feel-good factor, and can help to reduce mood swings and depression. Even a gentle session can help you to get a better night's sleep, while increasing your strength and postural awareness helps you to avoid injury.

'I've been doing yoga on and off for several years to tone and balance my body. When I haven't done any stretching for a few days I notice how stiff I've become, mentally as well as physically. I get tired more quickly now that I'm pregnant and sometimes I'm too lazy to bother after working all day, but then I can't ease my back or fasten my shoes in the way that I can when I practise regularly. I feel so much better when I make myself practise.'

Sally (37), 28 weeks pregnant

Your body has many physical changes to accommodate during pregnancy, so moderate, low-impact exercise is more suitable than competitive sport or activities where you risk overstretching or have to work hard to keep up. Most women are able to adapt their usual activities, but ask your coach, teacher or doctor for advice if you are in any doubt.

In general, it is better to continue with a familiar sport or activity rather than trying something completely different during pregnancy. If you do try a new form of exercise, make sure that your instructor knows you are pregnant and is able to advise you. If you feel you are generally fit, you may want to improve your flexibility or strength by doing some of the exercises on pages 64–75.

Strength, suppleness and stamina are important when you are pregnant (see pages 14–15). Strong muscles support and protect ligaments that are softened by hormones. Suppleness allows your body a full range of mobility so that you can move with less effort and adopt advantageous positions when you are giving birth. Stamina provides the sustained energy you need to cope with the demands of pregnancy or a long labour.

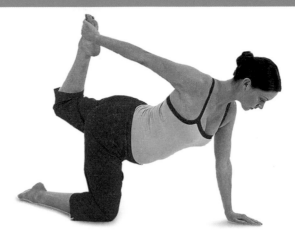

Above *Low-impact exercise such as yoga is more suitable than competitive sport while pregnant.*

Grades of exercise

The table below gives a rough idea of what ten popular forms of exercise can contribute to the individual elements of fitness when performed actively (a brisk walk, for example, not a stroll). The more stars, the greater the contribution.

	Strength	Stamina	Suppleness
Aerobics	**	***	***
Athletics	***	***	**
Badminton	**	**	***
Cycling	***	****	***
Dancing	**	****	***
Jogging	**	****	**
Swimming	****	****	****
Tennis	**	**	***
Walking	**	***	*
Yoga	**	**	****

Where to start

If your job and lifestyle are sedentary and you take no regular exercise, you will benefit greatly from regular gentle activity. Look for opportunities to walk instead of driving or using public transport. If you work on the upper floor of a building, instead of taking the lift walk down the stairs at first, then move on to climbing them. Within a short period you will start to feel more energetic and less tired at the end of the day, and you can progress to moderate exercise as your pregnancy advances.

If you are reasonably active but want to improve your fitness, try to fit in three 15- to 20-minute sessions of moderate exercise each week. You could buy a pregnancy exercise video or look for details of special classes for pregnancy on the noticeboard at your local leisure centre or hospital. Before joining a general exercise class, make sure that the teacher knows you are pregnant.

If you take part in competitive games, or sports that involve rigorous training or tempt you to push yourself, talk to your coach about the appropriate level of training. You may need to ease up or take special precautions. It is very unwise to strive to win, to finish a routine when you are exhausted or to push yourself to the point of being more than a little breathless.

Walk to fitness

Regular walking strengthens your legs, improves your flexibility and is easy to monitor. It provides good aerobic exercise, helping your lungs to take in more oxygen with less effort and increasing your stamina. If you do not generally take much exercise,

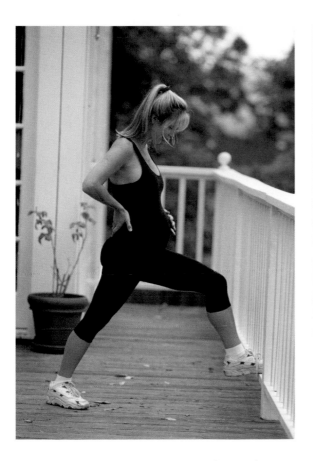

Safe pulse rate

Whatever your activity, you can check that you are exercising within safe limits by finding your maximum safe pulse rate in beats per minute. Subtract your age from 220 and multiply the result by 0.6 for the lower end of your range, and by 0.85 for the upper end.

Age	Pulse Rate	Age	Pulse rate
18	121–171	33	112–158
19	120–170	34	111–158
		35	111–157
20	120–170	36	110–156
21	119–169	37	110–155
22	118–168	38	109–154
23	118–167	39	108–153
24	117–166		
25	117–165	40	108–153
26	116–164	41	107–152
27	115–164	42	106–151
28	115–163	43	106–150
29	114–162	44	105–149
		45	105–148
30	114–161	46	104–147
31	113–160	47	103–147
32	112–159		

you will soon see an improvement in fitness if you walk for 20 minutes three times a week and keep a record of your pulse rate.

To do this, walk for ten minutes, and then check your pulse rate. If you find it is near the lower end of your range (see box), your speed is about right; if not, slow your pace down. As your fitness improves, your pulse rate will go down while you walk at the same speed or maintain the same level of activity.

For all forms of exercise, some authorities suggest that during pregnancy an upper pulse rate of 140 is desirable, regardless of age.

Above If you aren't used to walking, it might be an idea to stretch gently before you start (see pages 62–63).

Exercise safely

You might want to avoid sports such as skiing or horse-riding, where there is a risk of accidental injury, but in general most activities can be continued during pregnancy provided you listen to your body and make sensible adjustments.

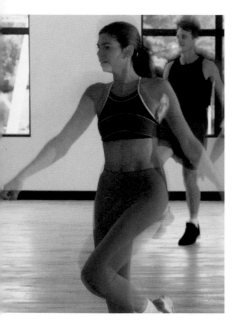

Above *If you continue with aerobics while pregnant, you may need to take it more gently to avoid strain.*

Opposite *Increasing postural awareness through exercise can help you to avoid injury during pregnancy.*

For example:
- Tell your yoga, aerobics, keep fit or dance teacher that you are pregnant, so that you can ease up to avoid strains.
- Jog on grass in trainers that prevent jarring.
- Use an exercise bike, or cycle on quiet roads rather than down mountains.
- When you play tennis or badminton, ask your partner to send shots you can return with ease.

Swimming provides excellent exercise, increasing strength, stamina and suppleness. However, arching your back to keep your head out of the water and kicking in breaststroke may make your back and pelvic ligaments ache. Change your leg movement if you feel any pain in your groin after swimming breaststroke, or use backstroke or front crawl to avoid strain.

If you have a disability or a chronic condition such as asthma or diabetes, or you are very overweight or unfit, you may want to ask your doctor if there is anything specific you should bear in mind before starting an exercise programme.

Safety guidelines
- If you have had a recent miscarriage, have high blood pressure, or you smoke and your BMI (see pages 42–43) is over 30, check with your doctor before starting an exercise programme.
- Your pulse rate should stay under 140 and your temperature under 38°C (100°F).

- Keep strenuous activity to a maximum of 15 minutes per session. Avoid it in hot or humid weather, or if you feel unwell.
- If you are a competitive athlete, discuss the appropriate level of training with your coach.
- In some cases, you may need to take up a more moderate form of exercise that you can continue to enjoy throughout pregnancy.
- Never strive to win, finish a routine when you are exhausted or push yourself to the point of being more than a little breathless.
- Avoid anything that causes strain or feels uncomfortable.
- Seek advice from your doctor or midwife if you have any unusual symptoms.

Q A few weeks ago I started to feel an ache in my groin and now I get pain around my pubic bone. Should I be concerned?

A The three separate bones that make up your pelvis are connected by ligaments that stabilize the joints as you move. During pregnancy hormones soften the ligaments, making your pelvis less stable than usual. Pelvic aches are common in pregnancy, but pain in the joints is not normal.
Warning signs that your joints are under stress include things like discomfort while walking, climbing stairs or turning over in bed. By recognizing these you can try to avoid movements or activities that cause the discomfort, to prevent the condition from getting worse. If your pelvic joints ache, for example, avoid stretching your legs apart, and swimming if the discomfort persists.

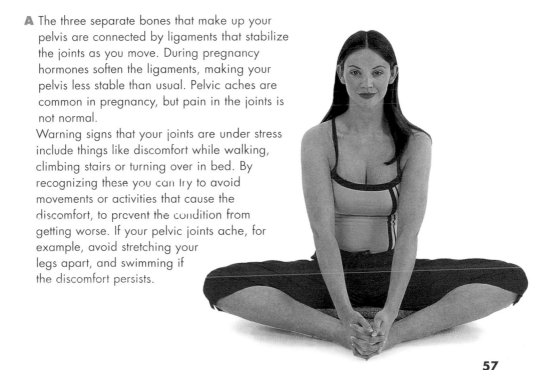

Stretching in pregnancy

Some women are naturally supple, while others have more

stamina or strength. Regular stretching will enable you to get to

know what your body is capable of and help you to accept both

its abilities and its limitations. If you stretch every day you should

notice an improvement in flexibility within a week or two, and

with practice you will gain the confidence to maximize your own

potential. You do not need to compete with anyone else.

Below Regular
stretching can
improve flexibility,
but make sure you
take it at your
own pace.

Stiff muscles feel uncomfortable when stretched, but the sensation feels 'right', not painful. A muscle pushed beyond its normal range of movement feels different from one that is simply stiff. During pregnancy it is easy to overstrain, so take care to keep all your movements within your own capability and control.

Improve your flexibility gradually, at your own pace and following the general safety advice given on pages 56–57. If you have any doubts about starting an exercise programme (a previous back or neck injury, for example) ask your doctor for advice. Stretching can improve some conditions, but it is always wise to check.

The more you practise, the fitter and more supple you will become. A marathon session that leaves you exhausted followed by a gap of several days is less beneficial than short, frequent sessions that become a way of life.

Keeping up the sessions

It is all too easy to start an exercise programme with great enthusiasm, only to fall by the wayside when other

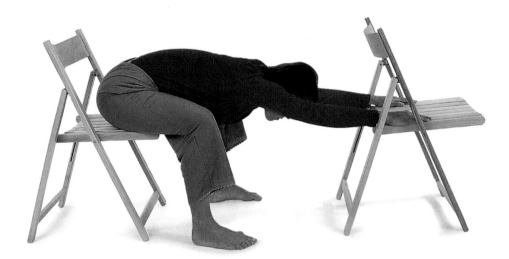

things take over or you feel tired, so it is worth finding the time of day that will work best for you to set aside for practice sessions. You'll probably find this practice time becomes a little oasis in the hurly-burly of your daily life.

- You could get up 20 minutes earlier for a stretching session to set you up calmly to face the rest of the day, or make it part of your wind-down routine, finishing with a warm, relaxing bath before bed.
- If you wake regularly in the middle of the night and cannot get back to sleep, you could practise for 20 minutes to calm your mind.
- You may wish to ask your partner to help, or team up with a friend or neighbour who is also pregnant to keep up regular sessions.
- If you already have other children, persuade them to join in – children tend to be naturally more flexible than adults and they often find stretching exercises fun.

If you ask for help to increase a stretch, guide your exercise partner so that he or she never apply more pressure than is comfortable and stop as soon as you give the word. Stretching beyond your comfort limit could be harmful.

Above *Always be guided by your body, and avoid anything that feels uncomfortable. It is easy to overstrain muscles during pregnancy.*

Exercise programme

The exercises on pages 62–75 are designed to stretch and tone your whole body, and are safe and easy to perform throughout pregnancy. If you practise you will become stronger, more supple, able to move gracefully and carry your pregnancy more comfortably. During labour you will be able to adopt positions that maximize the room in your pelvis, so that your baby can pass through it more easily.

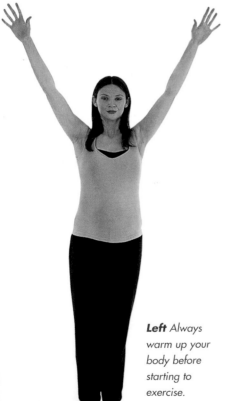

Left Always warm up your body before starting to exercise.

With any exercise programme during pregnancy start gently, build up slowly and always stop if you feel tired. Warm up first, cool down afterwards and drink plenty of fluids. Where a number of repetitions is not stated, use your judgment. Work to your maximum capability, which may vary from day to day, depending on how you feel and your stage of pregnancy. Keep your movements smooth and within your comfortable range.

Holding a pose for some length of time helps to increase stamina, but when you are pregnant a more 'fluid' approach is preferable, so that you maintain good circulation. Aim to hold each position for anything from a few seconds up to a few minutes. You can supplement these exercises with walking or swimming for extra stamina and all-round fitness.

If you are experienced at stretching, practise these exercises dynamically, moving smoothly from one position to another, almost like a dance. If you are new to it, relax into each position and try to be aware of the total effect on your body. This will help

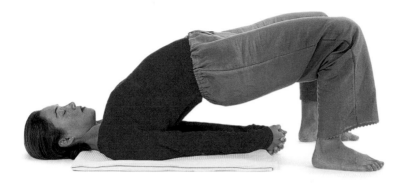

you to centre yourself, still your mind and relax more deeply – and is also an excellent preparation for giving birth.

Five steps to getting fitter

1 Warm up your muscles with a few gentle stretches (see pages 62–63), to music if you like.

2 Work on the basic exercises for your pelvic area (pages 66–67).

3 Work through the other exercises (pages 68–75). Vary them during the week, but try to do at least one exercise for each part of your body.

4 Think consciously about your posture during each exercise.

5 Finish each session with cool-down exercises (see pages 62–63) and relaxation (see pages 84–87). Relax as deeply as possible for as long as you can, then get up slowly.

Listen to your body

- Never force your body in any way – the key for stretching is little and often.

- If an exercise feels too strenuous, makes you light-headed or causes any other problem, leave it out.

- If you feel tired or under the weather, stop exercising until you feel better.

- If you cannot complete a session, just do as much as you feel able.

Above Exercising your body makes you more aware of its needs and unique abilities.

Warm up and cool down

Warming up increases your circulation, enables you to perform the exercises more effectively and helps to prevent injury to cold or stiff muscles. After a lengthy or intense exercise session, cooling down rather than stopping suddenly can prevent post-exercise stiffness.

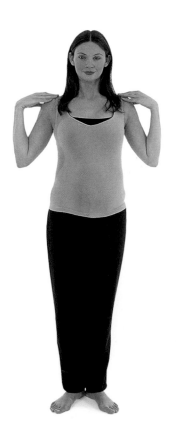

A warm up routine should gently increase your pulse rate, the rate and depth of your breathing and your muscle temperature. It can take almost any form, from climbing stairs to jogging on the spot; but wherever possible it should relate to the form of exercise to follow – in this case, stretching or increased flexibility.

This routine takes only a few minutes and can be used for both warming up and cooling down. Stand in a relaxed manner, with your feet slightly apart. Repeat each movement several times, keeping it slow and controlled.

1 Look towards your left shoulder, then sweep your chin down and around until you are looking towards your right shoulder, then back again.

2 Put your hands on your shoulders (left). Sweep your elbows in circles, then stretch out your arms and circle them.

3 Put your hands on your hips. Keeping your hips pointing forwards, twist your upper body to one side, then the other.

4 Drop your arms to your sides. Slide one hand down your leg without twisting your body. Repeat on the other side.

5 Using your pelvis, make circular movements in both directions (below).

6 Lunge forwards gently to stretch your calf and thigh muscles. Repeat with the other leg.

7 Extend one leg sideways to stretch your inner thigh. Repeat with the other leg.

8 Lift one leg, circle your foot at the ankle, then stretch it up and down. Repeat with the other foot. If necessary, use a wall for balance.

Caution

A systematic 'Cooling Down' routine can help eliminate the waste products produced by exercise, thereby increasing its effectiveness. Use this same routine to cool down, perhaps in reverse order.

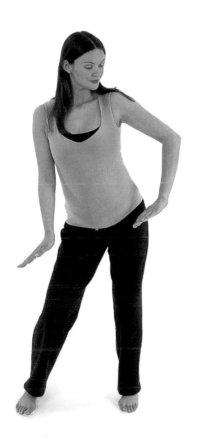
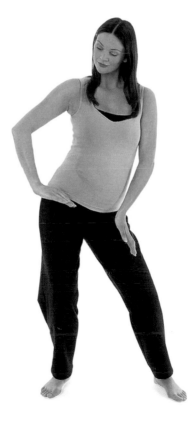

Inner thighs and lower back

If you are used to sitting on chairs rather than on the floor, you may be uncomfortable in positions that expand your pelvic ligaments to make giving birth easier, because the muscles of your inner thighs have shortened and your knees are stiff. These two stretches help to address this.

Caution

Avoid these stretches if you experience any pain in your groin, or in the area around your pubic bone.

Forward stretch

1 Sit with your back straight and stretch your legs as wide apart as is comfortable. Lift up from the waist to lengthen and widen your back.

2 Lean gently forward from the hip, keeping your back straight and pushing your heels away from you. Feel the stretch in your back, thighs and calves.

Benefits Lengthens the muscles in your inner thighs and increases the suppleness of your lower back.

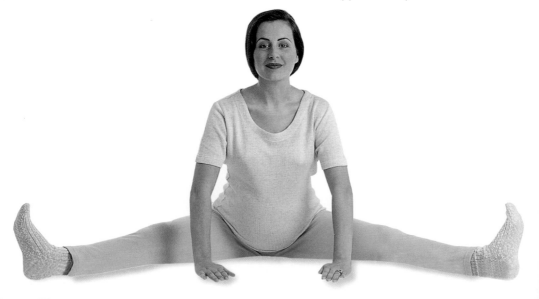

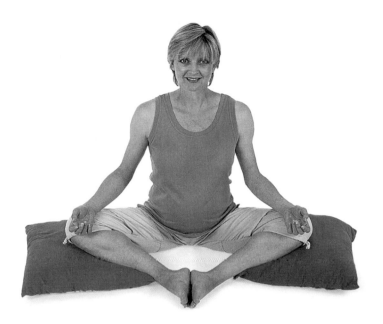

Tailor

1 Sit on the floor with your back against the wall. Lengthen your back and widen your shoulders.

2 Put the soles of your feet together and bring them close up to your body.

3 Rest your forearms on your knees and consciously relax your inner thigh muscles. You may wish to rest your thighs on cushions on the floor either side of you. Breathe down into your abdomen, emphasizing the 'out' breath.

Benefits Lengthens the adductor muscles in your inner thighs to release stiffness.

Caution

If your back is not against a wall, make sure you keep your spine straight and not slumped.

Pelvic mobility

If you are supple in the waist and pelvic area, you will be able to move more easily during late pregnancy and your baby will feel lighter to carry. These three exercises increase the suppleness of your pelvic area while toning and strengthening your lower back and abdominal muscles.

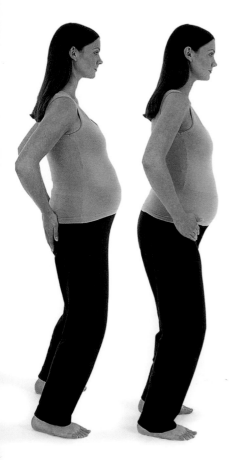

Pelvic rock

1 Stand with your feet apart and your knees slightly bent. Tighten your buttock muscles and tuck your 'tail' (the base of your spine) under.

2 Release your buttocks and swing your pelvis gently backwards. Tilt your pelvis backwards and forwards in a slow rhythm.

3 Using your waist muscles, tilt your pelvis from side to side.

4 Try both these movements with your knees straight instead of bent.

Benefits Strengthens your lower back and eases backache.

Caution

Make sure the movement uses your pelvis, not your legs or upper body.

Pelvic rotation

1 Put the two pelvic rock movements (left) together, so that you rotate your pelvis in one direction, then the other.

2 Try the rotation with your legs straight, then bent. Make the movement with your hips, not your legs.

Benefits Loosens your pelvis so that you can move more easily.

Pear-drop

1 Kneel on a cushion and lean forwards onto a birth ball, bean bag or chair, with a pillow placed on the seat. Keep your back horizontal.

2 Rock and rotate your pelvis in this position, then make an oval or pear-shaped movement, moving your whole body slowly and rhythmically.

Benefits Mobilizes your pelvis and can be very comforting during labour when your contractions are strong.

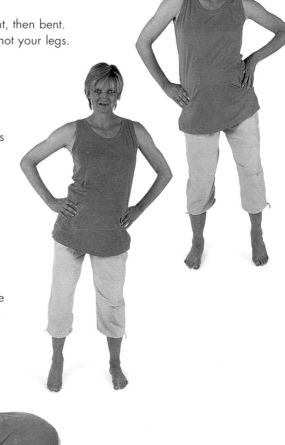

Upper body

Suppleness in your upper body helps to prevent unnecessary aches and pains. Strong shoulders and arms make lifting, carrying and changing position easier, especially in late pregnancy or if you are recovering from a caesarean section. The first two exercises strengthen your muscles and release tension in your neck and shoulders; the third strengthens the pectoral muscles on your chest wall, which help to support your breasts.

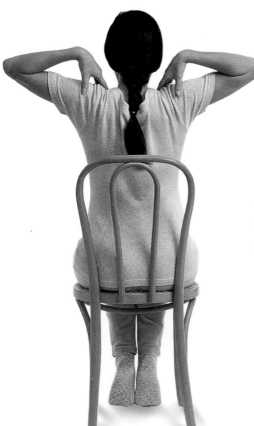

Neck and shoulders

1 Sit up straight on an upright chair, with your hands on your shoulders.

2 Lengthen and widen your back, then sweep your elbows around in wide circles. Feel the stretch across your shoulders and upper back.

Benefits Releases tension in your neck and shoulders.

Catherine wheels

1 Sit or stand with your arms stretched out to either side and your fists clenched.

2 Rotate your arms quickly in small circles, and then more and more slowly as you make ever-wider circles.

3 When you reach the widest stretch possible, gradually return to small, fast circles.

Benefits Strengthens your arms and helps to ease shoulder stiffness.

Pectorals

1 Stand with your feet hip width apart and your shoulders relaxed. Lengthen and broaden out your back.

2 Grasp your forearms just above your wrists and lift your arms to shoulder height.

3 Without loosening your grip or letting your arms drop, push your hands towards your elbows in small jerks. Feel your breasts move with each little push. Repeat 20 times.

Benefits Strengthens your arms and the pectoral muscles on your chest wall.

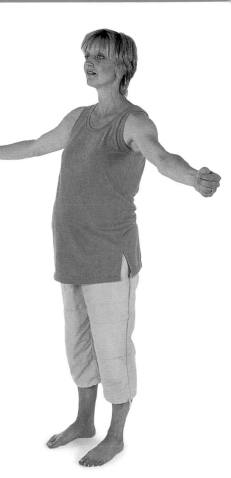

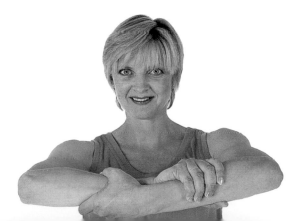

Lower body

These exercises tone and strengthen your abdomen, back and buttock muscles to improve your posture, help support your baby and reduce backache. Repeat each exercise 6–12 times, stopping if your muscles begin to tire.

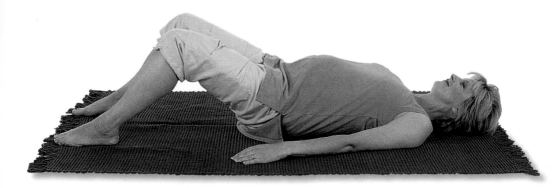

Caution

Avoid lying on your back if it makes you light-headed, or if you suffer from heartburn or high blood pressure.

Leg sliding

1 Lie on your back with your knees bent and your feet hip width apart.

2 Press your back to the floor and slowly slide your feet along the floor away from you. Use your abdominal muscles to keep your back firmly against the floor. When it starts to arch, bring your feet back up to the starting position.

3 If you are uncomfortable lying on your back, stand with your feet slightly apart and your back to a wall. Using your abdominal muscles, press your back into the wall. Hold the position for a few seconds, then release slowly.

Benefits Tones your abdominal muscles without straining them.

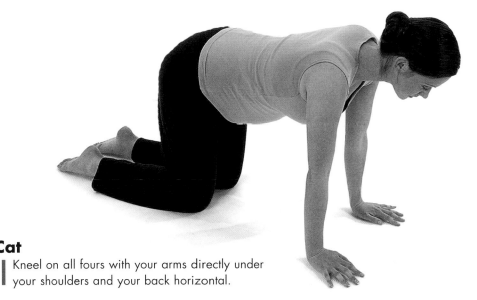

Cat

1 Kneel on all fours with your arms directly under your shoulders and your back horizontal.

2 Without arching your back at all, tighten your buttock muscles to tilt your pelvis under, then release them.

3 Keeping your back straight and your thighs and arms upright, bend at the waist and look towards your left hip. Repeat, looking towards your right hip.

Benefits Tones your lower back, buttock and abdominal muscles while helping to improve your pelvic flexibility.

Leg strength

Your legs will strengthen naturally to support the added weight of your baby, but as pregnancy advances you may find it increasingly difficult to get up from a chair or climb stairs easily. Strong thigh muscles make these everyday exertions easier. They also enable you to use upright positions during labour and to move more easily if you are recovering from a caesarean section.

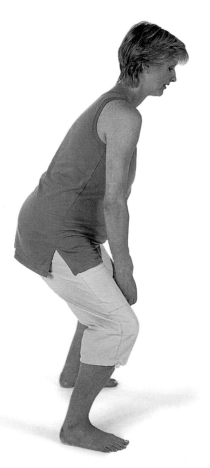

Monkey

1 Stand with your feet hip width apart. Lengthen and widen your back.

2 Drop into a shallow squat, bending your ankles, knees and hips together. Relax your shoulders so that your arms hang loosely in front of you.

3 Check that your back is straight, your neck is perfectly aligned with your spine and your weight is evenly distributed through your feet. If your centre of gravity is too far forward or too far back you will feel less comfortable. Hold the position until your legs begin to tire.

Benefits Strengthens your thighs and makes you aware of how your joints work in harmony to produce an economical movement that feels 'right'. Use this basic movement to pick up things from the floor or take food out of the fridge, instead of bending with straight legs or a rounded back.

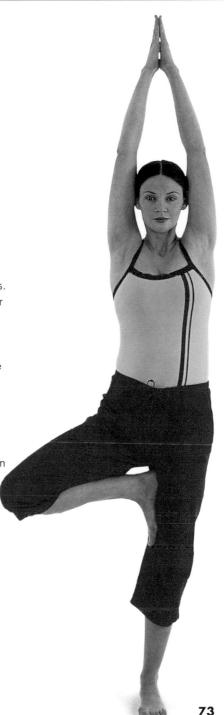

Top tips

To keep your balance, fix your eyes on a point across the room. Keep your palms together and close to your chest (in a prayer position) at first if you find it easier.

Tree

1 Lengthen your back and widen your shoulders. Shift your weight onto one leg, bend the other knee and rest the foot against your lower leg (or your thigh if your prefer).

2 Rotate your knee out to the side, making sure your spine and neck are aligned. Relax your shoulders, look straight ahead, and stretch your arms wide or press your hands together, palm to palm. Repeat with the other leg.

Benefits This adaptation of a classic yoga position strengthens your legs, opens your pelvis and improves your sense of balance.

Circulation and pelvic floor

During pregnancy hormones cause your artery and vein walls to relax, while extra blood circulates around your body to supply oxygen to your baby and remove waste products. The following exercise helps to maintain good circulation.

Foot work

1 Sit on the floor with your back supported. Rotate your ankles anti-clockwise, then clockwise.

2 Flex your feet alternately up towards your nose, then down to the floor, as though you were working foot pedals.

3 Repeat each movement until your muscles begin to tire.

Benefits Improves circulation to help avoid discomforts such as cramp, varicose veins or haemorrhoids.

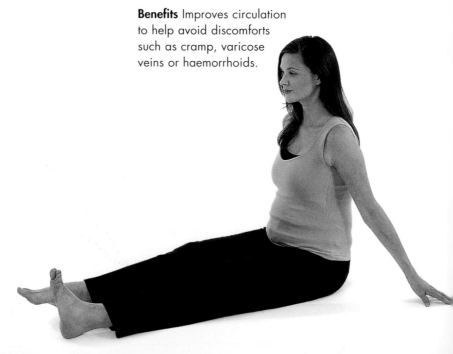

Pelvic floor

Your pelvic floor supports your uterus and controls the openings to your front and back passages. Strong muscles improve your sex life, prevent leaking when you cough or laugh, and help to turn your baby's head so that it passes more easily through your pelvis when you are giving birth.

Start to tone your pelvic floor as early as possible in pregnancy, so that it performs its work more effectively. The sensations may be harder to feel later on when the muscles have to work against an increasing weight.

1 Slowly tighten and release the muscles between your legs six to eight times, repeating several times a day. Try it standing, kneeling or lying down, until you find the most effective position.

2 To increase your control, imagine your pelvic floor is a lift and draw the muscles up in stages, stopping at each level. Let them out in stages (this is more difficult!). Start with two levels and progress to six or seven as the muscles become more and more responsive.

3 Distinguish and then work the muscles around your front and back passages separately. First tighten and release them, then try the 'lift' exercise with each group.

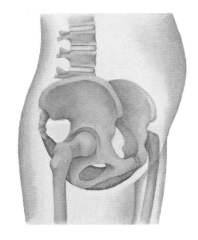

Above *Your pelvic floor provides a hammock that supports your internal organs and your growing baby.*

Caution

Avoid lying on your back if it makes you light-headed, or if you suffer from heartburn or high blood pressure.

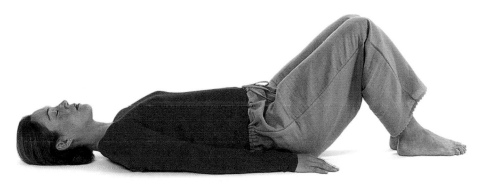

saving energy

- Use your body well

- Body work

- In labour

- Learn to relax

5

- Deep relaxation

- Conserve your energy

- Complementary therapies to help you relax

Use your body well

Exercise increases your strength, suppleness and postural awareness, so that you can lift things and move in a way that does not cause you injury. Another effective way to avoid aches and save energy is to use your body well. This means consciously avoiding movements that place unnecessary strain on it.

'I learned how to use my body well at antenatal classes. We used the 'monkey' (see page 72) for sitting down and standing up, and my ability to spring comfortably and lightly to my feet surprised and impressed me. It helped my posture in the run-up to the birth. You have to stop and think and it's easier not to bother, but when I feel heavy or weary, just thinking about a movement before putting it into action calms me and I feel in control again.'

Dawn (32), 39 weeks pregnant.

The manner in which you use your body affects everything you do. When you use it well your bones, muscles and ligaments interact perfectly. They share the extra weight, naturally correct your balance, and stabilize joints and ligaments affected by softening hormones. As a result, every activity takes less effort; you feel more comfortable during pregnancy, labour is easier and you feel better after the birth. Using your body effectively and with the least effort takes practice, but it is learning for life.

During pregnancy your centre of gravity changes and the curve in your spine increases naturally as your baby grows. You feel different. The balance and alignment of your body is constantly adjusted by your postural reflex, a complex mechanism that helps you to know subconsciously where your body is in space, so that you can move freely without having to look at your feet or hold on to things.

Changing habits

Many of the common aches and pains that are associated with pregnancy are the result of poor habits. For example:
• You are more likely to suffer from backache if your posture is poor, because your ligaments can become strained.

• Sitting or standing badly makes heartburn and breathlessness more likely: your stomach and lungs are already restricted by your uterus and slumping down in a chair or standing with rounded shoulders puts extra pressure on them.
• Lifting badly can strain the ligaments that stabilize your spine.

Most people take their body for granted until it shrieks in protest. When you are pregnant, it demands attention sooner – good habits can be easier to learn as you get faster feedback.

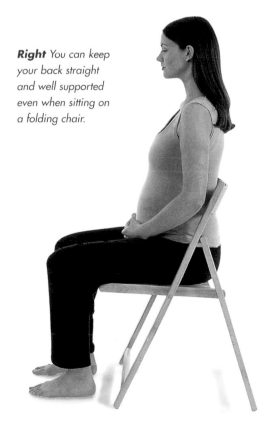

Right You can keep your back straight and well supported even when sitting on a folding chair.

Body basics

• **Consciously lengthen and widen your back, instead of rounding your shoulders and squashing your internal organs.**

• **If you lift a child or a heavy bag, bend your knees and hold the weight close to your body. Transfer it from place to place by moving your feet instead of twisting.**

• **To help prevent backache, hold your spine with a small natural curve at the waist and your head up and forward, not thrust out or pulled back.**

• **Wear comfortable shoes with low or medium heels. High, narrow heels may tilt your pelvis, throwing your weight onto the balls of your feet.**

Body work

When you use your body well, it feels lighter and every movement is easy and comfortable. At first you may move badly without thinking. Correcting your posture may feel slightly awkward, because muscles become weak and tire easily when you are not accustomed to using them. However, if you persevere they will quickly strengthen, and with practice good movements will become a habit.

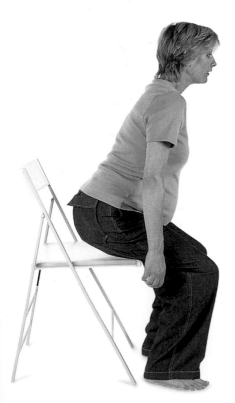

Standing well

1 Imagine your back is long and wide, while your head floats freely at the top of your spine, like a table tennis ball on a jet of water. Notice how much better it feels without that crunched-up sensation under your ribs.

2 Take off your shoes and feel your weight evenly distributed over the soles and heels of your feet.

Getting up from a chair

1 Stop and think about the movement you are going to make. Lengthen and widen your back, then shift your weight to the edge of the chair and plant your feet firmly.

2 Lean forward slightly and get up smoothly, without letting your knees move towards each other or pushing yourself up with your hands. As you rise, think 'up' and lead with your head. If you like, imagine being pulled upwards by a golden thread attached to your head. Notice how much lighter the movement feels.

Turning over and getting out of bed

1 When you turn over in bed during the night, keep your knees together and roll from your side to your back and then to the other side.

2 Roll to face the edge of the bed and bend your knees a little. Push up with your arms and swing your legs over the edge of the bed so that you are sitting upright. Get up as you would from a chair.

Lifting

1 Position yourself close to whatever you are going to pick up, such as a bag of shopping or your toddler, so that you can keep the weight near to your body.

2 Bend your knees, hips and ankles at the same time and keep your back straight but inclined, so that your thighs take the strain as you lift. Any form of exercise that helps to strengthen your thighs will make lifting easier (see 'Leg strength', pages 72–73).

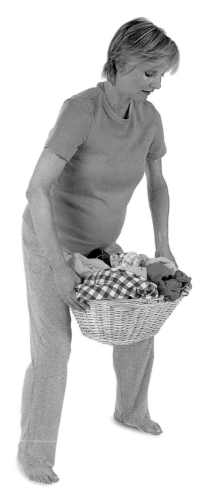

In labour

The way you use your body affects your comfort in labour just as much as during pregnancy. If you are supple and aware you will instinctively pick the right positions, and the more you are able to do so the easier your labour is likely to be.

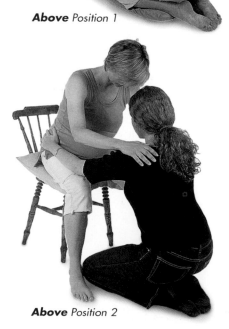

Above *Position 1*

Different positions can have different effects on the progress of labour:

- Upright positions enlist the aid of gravity, so standing, kneeling up, sitting or squatting tend to make the contractions stronger and more effective.
- Horizontal positions, such as kneeling on all fours or leaning forwards onto a birth ball, can slow down labour or ease backache.
- Lying on your side also tends to slow down labour, as it changes the forces of gravity. This may give you respite from extremely strong contractions and could also help your midwife to deliver your baby's head by controlling it as it emerges.

Gently rocking your pelvis when you are standing up, kneeling, sitting or lying down can be comforting in labour. If your progress is slow, you could try rocking your pelvis from side to side. Some midwives suggest climbing stairs sideways (facing the banister) to encourage your baby into a better position.

When you push your baby into the world, try to keep your pelvis free so that you can move in whatever way your body dictates. Lying on your back is not helpful, because your sacrum (the base of your spine) is fixed and cannot move. Leaning forward allows it to swing open, increasing the room in your pelvis by up to 30 per cent so that your baby has more space through which to pass.

Above *Position 2*

If`you semi-squat or kneel and lean onto your partner or the head of the bed, you enlist the help of gravity and can arch your back instinctively to straighten out the birth canal and make pushing easier.

Positions for labour

1 Sitting on the floor, spread your knees to make room for your bump and lean forward onto your partner.

2 Sit on a chair with your knees apart, leaning onto your partner.

3 Stand leaning onto your partner, the wall or a piece of furniture during contractions.

4 Kneel on all fours, or lean onto your partner or a birth ball.

5 Sit reversed on a chair padded with a pillow. Relax onto another pillow placed on the back of the chair.

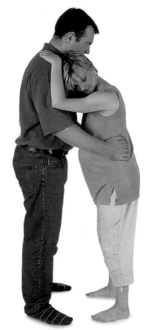

Above Position 3

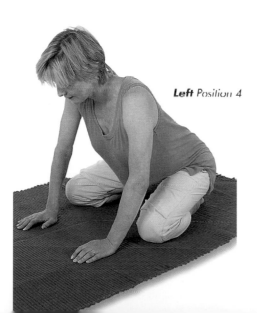

Left Position 4

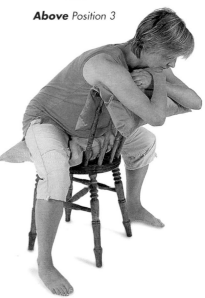

Above Position 5

Learn to relax

Relaxation is a skill that anyone can learn. It simply involves recognizing tension and consciously letting it go. Try this exercise every day for two weeks, keeping the sessions short (5–10 minutes each). With a little practice you will only need to check groups of muscles in order to stay relaxed.

Relaxation step by step

Sit in a comfortable chair or lie down, whichever you prefer.

1 Tighten up one leg as much as possible, notice what this feels like, then let go completely and feel the difference. Then tighten and release in turn: your other leg, lower back and buttock muscles, tummy muscles, shoulders, arms and hands, neck, jaw, cheeks, lips, eyes and finally your forehead.

Below A really comfortable position makes it much easier for you to relax your body completely.

2 Go around your body again. This time tighten each group of muscles very slightly, letting go as soon as you are aware of the feeling of tension.

3 Go around your body a third time, simply checking that each muscle group is completely relaxed. If not, release the tension. When you are fully relaxed, observe how gentle and quiet your breathing has become.

4 When the session is over, stretch, wriggle you fingers and get up slowly. Deep relaxation can lower your blood pressure and if you jump up suddenly you may feel dizzy or light-headed.

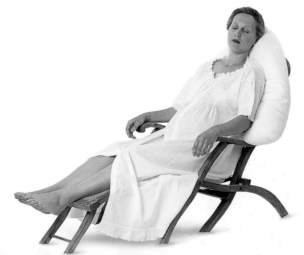

Breathing awareness

When you go about everyday tasks, or practise relaxation, you rarely think about breathing: your lungs expel used air and draw the next breath automatically. As your body becomes less relaxed, however, your breathing changes subtly. If you get really tense it becomes jerky – eventually you start to panic and gasp for air, so that you take in too much oxygen. This is called hyperventilation: you feel light-headed and experience a tingling sensation in your fingers. Being in this state reduces the amount of oxygen available to your baby and makes you feel awful.

Breathing and relaxation go hand in hand: when one changes, so does the other. If you breathe in a panicky, jerky fashion you will start to feel tense – notice the effect on your shoulders and arms. Equally, tensing your muscles deliberately while breathing gently is difficult, because your whole body wants to let go.

Breathing and relaxation during labour

Notice how you breathe when you are relaxed and, conversely, how relaxed you feel when you breathe gently. Staying relaxed during labour allows your uterus to work efficiently and makes the whole experience easier.

Aim to make your breathing as quiet and effortless and your muscles as relaxed as possible during labour. The secret is to recognize slight tension in your body or changes in your breathing at the earliest moment and then readjust them consciously before they have a chance to take hold.

Left Full chest breathing, which can be practised in this position with your partner, will help you to relax during labour. Relax consciously and aim your breathing at your partner's hands; he or she should feel a slight movement below your waist.

Deep relaxation

Once you are confident that you can relax at will, try these methods to help you relax more deeply. One or other of them may enable you to let go more easily, or may work better on certain occasions.

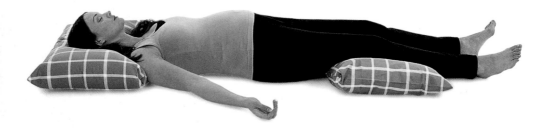

Above If you are not comfortable lying on your back, or if you suffer from heartburn or high blood pressure, use pillows to prop yourself up.

Special place

Choose a place that you already associate with feeling relaxed, indoors or out, real or imaginary. Visualize it vividly – what you can see, the sounds, the smells, the colours, the weather, the time of day and so on. Let your mind play freely, but try to place yourself in the scene, rather than as a bystander observing yourself from the outside.

Descending steps

Imagine standing at the top of a flight of ten steps. Descend slowly, counting from ten down. With each step, pause for a moment to let tension go, so that when you reach the bottom step – if not before – you are deeply relaxed.

Candle

Light a candle and sit where you can see it comfortably. You may like to use a floating candle in a bowl of water. Focus on the shape, colour and movement of the flame, the shadows cast, the candle itself and its container. Close your eyes and observe the reverse image on your retina. If your mind wanders, bring it gently back to the candle, consciously releasing the muscles of your face.

Sounds

In quiet surroundings, focus your attention on the sounds that enter the room. Identify each one and decide whether it is welcome or unwelcome. If your mind wanders off the task, gently bring it back and relax your face muscles. Many people relax best when listening to certain types of music, or to tapes of water, leaves rustling or bird song.

The pebble

Imagine that you are floating in the centre of a pool, the water supporting your body so that you almost feel part of it. There is no breeze; the water is quite still. Imagine a pebble dropped where your navel would be: ripples travel to the edges of the pool, taking tensions or troubles with them.

'I live life at breakneck speed and I was shocked by how much pregnancy slows you down. I got so overtired that I had difficulty sleeping and then I worried about not getting the sleep I needed for work. The more anxious I was the less I slept, until it became a vicious circle. My doctor told me to slow down and gave me two weeks off work. I bought a relaxation tape and had some reflexology sessions to get me back into a sleep routine. Now if I feel tired I go through my relaxation routine before stress gets a grip on me.'

Sally (41), 31 weeks pregnant

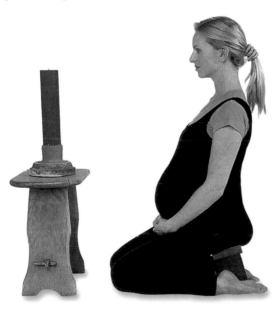

Left *Use a candle to help you relax more deeply.*

Conserve your energy

Everyone feels tired or needs an energy boost from time to time during pregnancy. There is no magic way to help you to feel on top of the world, but there are lots of little ways to help yourself enjoy the waiting months and they all add up.

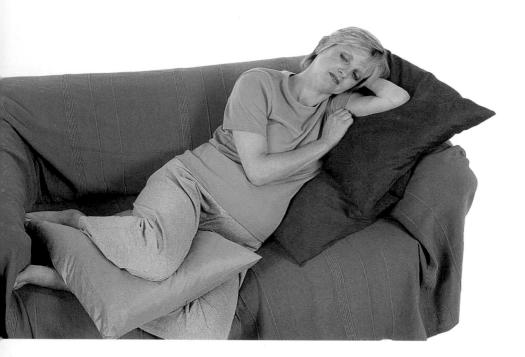

Above *Ensure that when you feel tired during the day, you take time to rest.*

Respect your body: it works overtime when you are growing a baby. It can be frustrating not to be able to do as much as usual, but this is a useful preparation for the constraints of having a new baby. If you are overworked or short of rest you can feel like a hamster in a tread wheel – all your energy drains away, and the harder you work the less you achieve.

Take time

Scurrying about burns more energy than moving along steadily, so pace yourself if you want to get through the day more easily.

- Plan ahead and write things down – remembering them takes mental energy.
- Pause before taking on a new commitment and consider how easily you can cope with it.
- If a task is not essential, finish it tomorrow – or the next day.

Eat regularly

Pregnancy is not the time to skip breakfast or shop through your lunch hour. You are likely to have more energy if you eat regularly to keep your blood sugar level up.

- Try eating your main meal at lunchtime and have a snack in the evening.
- Ask your partner to prepare the main meal.
- Save time by making a batch of sandwiches at the weekend and freezing them in plastic wrap to take to work, or to eat as soon as you get home.

Take a rest

When you feel tired during the day, try to stop and rest.

- Learn to 'power nap': relax completely for ten minutes (see pages 84–87).
- After lunch, have a nap or a rest with your feet up if you can, then make yourself get up and go for a brisk walk in the fresh air.
- If you are still working, a rest in your lunch hour may help you to feel fresher in the afternoon, or to socialize later in the day without falling asleep.
- Go to bed early at least once a week.
- Arrange with your partner to catch up on missed sleep by having at least one at the weekend, especially if you have small children or a demanding job.

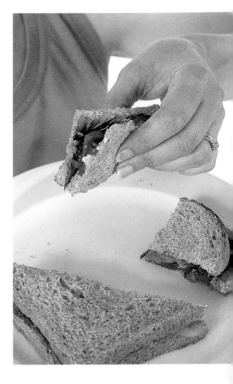

Above *To keep your energy levels high, it is important to eat regular healthy meals.*

Complementary therapies to help you relax

Many women use complementary therapies to enhance their general wellbeing and help them relax. Remedies are widely available over the counter in pharmacies and many can be used for self-treatment during pregnancy.

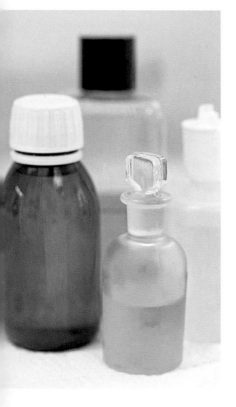

Above *Some aromatherapy oils can be used safely during pregnancy and can help you to relax.*

If you are not familiar with their use, or are unsure which remedy to choose or whether it is suitable for use during pregnancy, ask the pharmacist for advice. If you need individual advice or your condition does not respond to an off-the-shelf remedy, consult a qualified therapist.

Aromatherapy

Use the mild oils during pregnancy, mixing them where appropriate with a pure vegetable oil such as almond or grapeseed.

- For a massage, try one or two drops of lavender or chamomile Roman in 1 teaspoon (5ml) of almond oil.
- Try two drops each of the same oils in a room burner, or place one drop of lavender on your pillow at night.
- For a bath oil, mix two drops each of lavender and vetiver with a drop of valerian, and use two drops of this blend for a really relaxing soak.

Homeopathy

This works 'holistically', so you need to match the remedy to your individual characteristics and symptoms and follow the instructions on the pack. Avoid strong flavours such as peppermint toothpaste or coffee, as they impair the effectiveness of the remedies. Stop the treatment as soon as there is an improvement, but if it does not help or you keep repeating it, consult a qualified homeopath.

- If you cannot relax through worry, overwork or over-excitement, Kali. Phos. may help.
- If you are restless and irritable, try Chamomilla.
- When you cannot sleep because your mind churns round and round, try Coffea.
- If you are too tired to sleep, Cocculus may be more effective.

Medical herbalism

Make a herbal tea using a tea bag or a teaspoonful of dried herb per cup of boiling water. Leave it to stand for ten minutes and drink it on its own, or with milk and honey to taste.

- Try chamomile to relax your nervous system and your digestion.
- Lemon balm and linden blossom (lime flowers) help promote mental relaxation and have a calming effect on the body.
- A herbal infusion is more potent, contains more herb and is steeped for longer.
- To help you sleep, try leaving a handful of Californian poppy or elder flowers in 0.5 litre (1 pint) of boiling water for 30 minutes, then strain the liquid into a hot bath.
- Alternatively, make a similar bath infusion from hops or passion flowers.

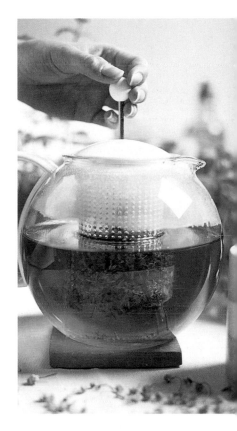

Above *Herbal teas are easy to make and have a calming effect on the body.*

'On the whole I love being pregnant – we didn't plan a large family, but somehow the babies just kept coming. I like taking responsibility for my own health. When I was expecting Heidi I thought I didn't need to make any effort, but by now I've learned that I need to be organized and to look after myself, or everyone suffers. I go to an exercise class partly to make sure I'm fit for the birth but also to enjoy sharing gossip with other pregnant women and to give some attention to this baby. When I feel low or frustrated I use my Bach flower remedies to take the edge off the stress and help me to get life in perspective again.'

Tanya (34), mother of Heidi (9), William (7), Cameron (4) and Gracie (22 months) and 32 weeks pregnant

Bach flower remedies

Bach flower remedies are used to treat emotional states rather than symptoms and many women use them to relieve stress. The best known is Rescue Remedy, a composite of five others: Star of Bethlehem for shock, Rock Rose for terror and panic, Impatiens for mental stress and tension, Cherry Plum for desperation and Clematis for feeling withdrawn or distant.

There are 38 individual Bach flower remedies, all widely available in healthfood stores and pharmacies.

- Try Aspen if you feel unable to relax because you are apprehensive.
- Use Olive if you have too much to do, no time to relax and no energy reserves.
- Vervain may help if you are frustrated by not being able to do all that you want to.
- White Chestnut is the remedy if you wake at night with your mind racing round obsessively.
- Hornbeam helps to combat mental exhaustion.

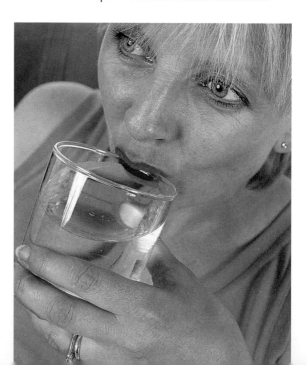

Right *Bach flower remedies, taken either on the tongue or in water, can be used to treat stress.*

Quick pick-me-ups

- Whiz a banana with some fresh orange juice in your blender, or with ice cream and milk, for a smooth and tasty drink that will give you a quick energy boost.

- Blend a glass of milk with 2 tablespoons (30ml) of natural yoghurt and a banana, or a glass of orange juice with six dried apricots (buy them pre-soaked) and a teaspoonful of honey. Add a teaspoon of brewer's yeast for extra vitamin B.

- Keep snacks like raisins, dried apricots or muesli bars within easy reach, to nibble when you need a lift. If you like chocolate, choose a bar that is at least 70 per cent cocoa solids – then you can comfort yourself that it is high in iron!

- A cup of peppermint tea with a 1cm (1/2in) chunk of fresh ginger root grated into it can be revitalizing. Tea and coffee reduce iron absorption, so drink water, fruit juice or herbal teas sometimes instead.

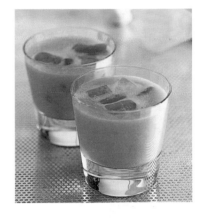

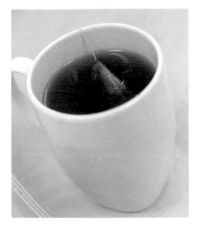

Right, above Mixing fresh fruit and juice can give your flagging energy levels a boost.

Right below Herbal teas are a good alternative to tea and coffee, which reduce iron absorption.

Index

Picture Credits

Octopus Publishing Group
Limited/David Jordan 20, 36, 37,
38, 39 bottom/Daniel
Pangbourne 1, 64, 68, 84/Emma
Peios 91/Peter Pugh-Cook 2, 5,
10, 11, 12, 13, 15, 17, 21, 24,
25, 26, 27, 31, 39 top, 53, 57,
58, 59, 60, 61, 62, 63 left, 63
right, 65, 66 left, 66 right, 67
top, 67 centre, 67 bottom, 69
top, 69 bottom, 70, 71, 72, 73,
74, 75, 79, 80, 81, 82 top, 82
bottom, 83 top, 83 bottom right,
83 bottom left, 85, 86, 87, 88,
89, 92/William Reavell 30, 32,
40/Gareth Sambidge 48, 90, 93
bottom/Karen Thomas 93 top
Photodisc 7, 8, 14, 16, 18, 22, 23,
44, 46, 49, 55, 56

Acknowledgements

I wish to acknowledge with gratitude
the work of Janet Balaskas, who first
inspired my interest in exercise
during pregnancy. Thanks also to the
thousands of pregnant women who
have attended my exercise classes
over the past twenty years and from
whom I have learned so much.

Executive Editor Jane McIntosh
Editor Joss Waterfall
Executive Art Editor Joanna Bennett
Designer Ginny Zeal
Senior Production Controller Jo Sim
Picture Librarian Jennifer Veall
Special Photography Peter Pugh-Cook
Stylist Aruna Mathur